D1500179

Hair Care for
MOTHERS OF
BIRACIAL
DAUGHTERS

A NEW SCIENTIFIC APPROACH
TO HAIR CARE

ShamBOOsie

Introduction

The Best Way to Use This Book for Maximum Effectiveness

In this book you will find the secrets I have used in the salon for over thirty years, and they work. If you really want to grow the most beautiful, healthy hair you have ever had, reading this book from cover to cover is required. Read every word on every page before you do anything else to your hair or try any of the recommendations of this book.

Consider this to be an educational guide to truly understanding how your hair works. What you will also find within these pages are the exact methods I've used in the salon for over thirty-four years successfully. Every product, formula, technique, and method of application has been tested a thousand times. If you will do exactly as the book teaches and don't add or omit *anything* I promise you will get the exact results promised in this book. You must completely trust **ShamBOOsie** and this book. I'm serious—if you want the promised results, you cannot add other products or your own ideas or omit or alter even a single concept.

This is not a "recipe book for hair"; it is a step-by-step Instructional Guide. In order to change the way you think about your hair care regimen, you must set aside all your own ideas. They haven't worked for you, and they never will, which is why you are reading this book. I care more about your hair than anyone you know, maybe even more than yourself. It is my total purpose to make this easier for you. You must be willing to trust the information I provide and make a commitment to follow the plan. **ShamBOOsie** will get you to where you want to be with your hair. Ask yourself whether what you are currently doing to your hair is working? If the answer is *no*, the information in this book is FOR YOU!

You can trust the recommended products because each product is excellent—among the best there is. I didn't write this book to be informative; I wrote it to truly help you with your hair. Don't be concerned about what anyone else will tell you—that's his or her opinion. This book is based totally on the theory, laws, science, and chemistry of cosmetology.

There's no need to keep this book pretty—Mark it up! Make notes for yourself in the book and use a marker to highlight the information that pertains to your specific hair-care issues. List the page number of the pages you need to find quickly on the blank page in the front of the book.

Why Are Quality Hair Care Products So Important?
The products mentioned in this book are the **Real Solutions to your very Real Hair Care Problems.** They are also the best remedy for preventing problems before they start. Go out and purchase ONLY the products you need and put this teacher to the test! You don't want to wait until you have problems to start caring for your hair; keep it as healthy as possible along the way as it GROWS.

This book is not about "conditioning your mind" but about great Hair Conditioners—the secret to the strength, health, SOFTNESS, beauty, and GROWTH of your hair. The most wonderful thing about the Superior Quality Hair Care Products is that they WORK. They will exceed the results achieved with anything else you have ever used to keep your hair healthy and strong.

Repetition Has Its Purpose:

To be *redundant* means to do or say the same thing over and over. Can you imagine how healthy your hair would be if you were redundantly diligent in shampooing and conditioning your hair every four to five days for four to six weeks? Remember, the purpose of this book is to teach you how to properly care for your hair so that you can grow a beautiful head of healthy hair. Repeating the most crucial pieces of information from time to time will ensure your success in learning how to properly care for your hair.

When you use the right products the right way, it will result in stronger, healthier, more beautiful, and longer hair every time. I have personally selected each product, so you can be confident it is the very best, but more importantly they will deliver. Specific hair care problems are addressed here by introducing EXACT Products and Exact application methods that produce EXACT results. Learn what each one is for and how to use it correctly, and then watch it do its job. Each product is the very best, and is very special and different from everything else in its individual category. All the formulas must be followed precisely to work.

It is my pleasure to share my findings of more than twenty-four years of research with you. Yes, you can grow and have beautiful hair; let me show you how.

SHAMBOOSIE—the name you can trust!

ShamBOOsie's Methodology

My methodology allows the hair to be **Chemically Relaxed *ONLY* *ONCE* during the life of the hair no matter how long the Hair GROWS.** The hair does GROW, even when chemically relaxing the hair every six to eight weeks. So, what exactly is **ShamBOOsie's Methodology?** It describes how everything about Black Hair works and how to care for it. It represents practical ideas and proven practices that include everything the woman of color will need to be successful in caring for, GROWING, and keeping her hair healthy, soft, strong, and so beautiful.

If you stay within the parameters and rules of ShamBOOsie's Methodology, the outcome will always be predictable. It is the best way to achieve perfection, and with it Real Hair GROWTH is inevitable! ShamBOOsie's Methodology features a perfect approach to caring for Black Hair, a *Wellness Approach*, one that will WORK every time, and hair products you can purchase at any local drug store that address each area of concern. The products are readily available on store shelves all over the country.

The Author believes that Black Women need to understand how their Hair Works to make CARING for their Hair Work the way it should. It's based on the chemistry of Black Hair and the way Black hair is supposed to work; it's the right way to do things every time without damaging the hair. In every area of CARING for their hair, Black Women want to know what to do, how to do it, and why it should be done. His Methodology incorporates an accurate concept for determining when the different stages are completed and ways that allow you to physically see the end results. If real GROWTH is your goal, then ShamBOOsie's Methodology is a commonsense approach to that end.

The Hair-Wellness Approach to Hair GROWTH is a collection of accurate techniques and steps used to identify, organize, and transform your hair-servicing requirements into an accurate application system that makes it simple to do. Once you refine the Application of the Chemical LYE Relaxer, the rest will be as easy as purchasing the right Hair Care Products and applying them on a regular basis. The research for this Hair Wellness Approach includes the method of a **"Hands-On Approach."** To answer every question required years of testing on many types of hair products. It was ShamBOOsie's **In-Salon, Hands-On Work** that brought about the amazing results and discoveries.

ShamBOOsie's Methodology is an accurate system of principles, procedures, and practices he has applied in the Salon for over thirty years. These procedures make CARING for Black Hair simple; it's a Step-by-Step Concept and a perfect fit for the layperson. Real Hair GROWTH is our goal and **the Methodology** is an effortless art to teaching the In-Home skills every black woman and mother needs to finally make some sense of her hair! It is the approach to achieving this goal. The idea here is to make sure it remains simple and to make sure it WORKS!

The methodology in this book supports the reader by presenting practical ideas and proven practices that include everything needed to be successful in Caring for, GROWING, and keeping her hair healthy, soft, and strong all along the way.

This Methodology is an In-Home seminar designed to provide practical solutions to difficult Hair Care problems and issues. It exposes participants to a set of accurate techniques, for systematically utilizing the laws, theory, and Science of Cosmetology. It helps her maintain the GROWTH, puts an end to the DRYNESS and Breakage, and ensures beautiful, manageable, healthy hair. **Now, finally, there's a Hair Wellness Approach to Hair Growth.** Too many Women of Color and Hairdressers alike go about handling Black Hair as if its Care and Health were less important than the cut, style, and the finished look. Then, of course, there is the money spent by black women on their hair, which is today hitting the $9 Billion mark! The Hair Wellness Approach is a designed discipline, which means all the difficulties have been removed, and the techniques, rules, and application procedures work and place the overall health of the hair at the top of the list.

ShamBOOsie's **Hair Wellness Approach to Hair Growth** is a commonsense yet scientific approach to the Care of Black Hair. This book is based on the Chemistry of your hair. If you are willing to purchase the needed High-End Hair Care Products, use them according to my methods of application, and if you are willing to do the work, you will get the desired results every time. It's the correct way, and it all makes sense.

ShamBOOsie purposely looked for a systematic approach, the *exact* products to effectively address the many Black Hair issues. I have created an easy-to-follow approach for performing each STEP in the process with confidence. Do it the same way each time and do it in a timely manner, and you will get the same results over and over again. Beautiful Healthy Hair and real GROWTH is our goal, and **ShamBOOsie's Methodology** is a strategy and approach to achieving this goal.

This book supports the reader in recognizing and understanding the meaning of words relevant to the subject of hair. It represents a collection of practical ideas that are proven practices, including everything the woman of color will need to do and know to be successful in GROWING her hair shoulder length or longer. It's about keeping the hair healthy, soft, and strong at the same time for its lifetime. This In-Home Torturing concept provides practical solutions to difficult Hair Care issues. The Author demonstrates techniques to GROW and maintain beautiful, manageable hair that are based on the theory of Cosmetology. It's a very real approach to getting it right every time.

I spend my time seeking a complete understanding of Black Hair— your hair—its Chemistry and Chemicals, and their effect on your hair. I must have a complete understanding of every product and Chemical needed to CARE for and protect your Hair. The Creator has given me the ability, skills, and the gifts needed to change the situation with Black Hair in this country. I have the gift of dyslexia, and I'm not referring to a reading disability, but the ability to see three and even four times as much of the world and what goes on here on the earth, with people, places, and things. The large manufacturers are taking advantage of black women, and I need to change this for you.

Everyone knows a black woman and many young Black Girls with Hair that is in POOR condition. For about 85 percent of Black Females in the country, their "GLORY" meaning their hair, is in crisis and needs help from someone knowledgeable enough, professional enough, and who cares enough to do something about it. I do care with all my heart.

Your hair should be groomed and worn in a tasteful and attractive manner. This is not the case for many Black Women and their

Daughters. If the hair is left on its own, it will soon become quite unattractive, which is the case with the Hair of millions of Women in this country. They simply don't know how to care for their hair or how to style it, which is part of the reason so few will do the necessary, yet time-sensitive, shampoos and CONDITIONERS the hair REALLY needs. This is what I teach, with simplicity. *Simply, follow my lead.*

In the initial phases of my mission to do something about this hair dilemma that most Black Women and their daughters are dealing with, I took the time to seek God's input. I asked for His guidance, and I prayed that He would help me write a book that would be truthful and on which readers could depend. I know that the Lord has His eye on everything I am doing with these books. It is He that has given me such a thorough and unique understanding of the subject of Black Hair and Hair in general.

God must always be the most important part of what I do. I would never ask the Lord to receive anything from me that was based on a lie. If I say that this concept really works, and it does not, then I am asking God to bless a lie. Just the thought of that scares me to death! In this book, I am demonstrating the correct way to apply a chemical relaxer without scalp burns and without severely damaging the hair. But I am using only words to describe the steps from start to finish. At best this will only create mental pictures. A Show-n-Tell, How-to DVD gives a whole new twist to the phrase a picture is worth a thousand words.

This **Methodology** is wrapped around the truth that seeing is believing. I fully intend for the reader to see real results—quickly! Otherwise I am asking God to take sin and bless it, and that's not what He does. You must be able to depend on my every word and believe that I can change everything you have been doing wrong with your hair and then teach you how to do things the right way—the way that really WORKS. The day I was on my way out to mail the first book to the publisher, my phone rang just as I touched the doorknob. It was my pastor. I told him I had written a book and was on my way out to mail it to the publisher. He said, let's pray about it, and he prayed for about ten minutes.

The first book has done amazing things, and this is what Christians call *confirmation*, which means it proves God has His hands on the books. My knowledge of hair and how to manage it is a gift from God, and I am hoping I can now use my gift for His glory. The books and the DVD I hope to produce soon are treasures I will store up in heaven. All that I do with these books will be for His glory, and He can give me back whatever portion He deems appropriate. So go ahead—IMAGINE MORE. It's time to Imagine More GROWTH than ever before. Imagine More Length, Healthier, Stronger, Softer, and more Beautiful hair than ever before. Place all your faith in God and step out on it, and Imagine More—it's time!

About the Author

Certification: A Certified Master Hair Instructor of Advance Techniques and Licensed in the State of New Jersey, with over thirty years in the industry. He has both a Cosmetology License and Instructor's License. Author of *Beautiful Black Hair: REAL Solutions to REAL Problems.* The first **Hair Care** book ever based on the Laws, Trichology (the Study of Hair) Science, Theory, and the Chemistry of Black Hair,—the way your HAIR really works.

The Science and the Chemistry of hair will always dictate! **Not ShamBOOsie.** You know what they say about opinions? They are like Eyeballs, and everybody's got at least one! This is the only Hair CARE book ever written for Women of Color and their Daughters that has any chance of helping them get it right!

ShamBOOsie has provided his professional Healthy Hair services for over thirty years, creating and replicating Hair CARE Solutions that take Hair CARE for Women of Color to the next level."

- Certified Master Hair Instructor of Advance Techniques - Licensed in the State of New Jersey
- Licensed Cosmetologist, Hair GROWTH, and Healthy Hair Specialist
- Master Hair Designer, and Chemical Application Specialist
- Certified Color Master – trained by Clairol Professional
- Creator of the "Let's Talk Hair" Seminar
- Creator of The 24 Month Hair GROWTH Timetable

Beautiful Black Hair

- Creator of A more Comfortable and Safer Way Relax Your Hair, without Breakage or Scalp Burns—Ever!
- Creator of The Hair Wellness Approach to Hair Growth – a NEW approach to Hair CARE teaching series.
- Author: *Beautiful Black Hair: REAL Solutions to REAL Problems.* The book was written based on the Theory of Cosmetology and the Laws and Science Trichology, the Study of Hair, and knowledge of the way your HAIR really works. The Science Dictates! Not **ShamBOOsie** or Cathy and any of her opinions. This is the only Hair CARE book ever written for Women of Color and their Daughters.

I Write Because I Love Your Hair!

I simply wanted to find a way to help you get hair care RIGHT. It's called **the Hair Wellness Approach to Hair GROWTH** because it's based on the **LAWS, THEORY, SCIENCE, and CHEMISTRY of Your Hair and Cosmetology!** I promise you that all the information you'll find in my books is as close to Scientific Accuracy as possible. The Science of **"Black Hair"** is an exact study, which means that it is a dependable study, and the results are as near to a perfect way of managing your hair and giving you positive results.

How to Get Your Hairdresser to Work with You

Having you Chemical Relaxer services managed properly is the most important aspect of Caring for and managing your hair and your daughter's hair. You and your Hairdresser will need to learn ShamBOOsie's Method of Application. If for some reason you prefer not to learn to Master the Art of Applying the Chemical LYE Relaxer with No Scalp Burns Ever, take this book (and DVD when it's ready,) to your Hairdresser and ask her to take a little time and look over ShamBOOsie's Hair Wellness Approach to Relaxing Black

Hair. Show her the kind of money you are willing to spend with her salon.

ShamBOOsie's challenge here is solving the 250-Year-Old-Hair-GROWTH Mystery! The reason this incredible undertaking is referred to as **Solving the 250-Year-Old-Hair-GROWTH Mystery.** Women of Color just can't get their hair to GROW or stay in place long enough to GROW because they lose their hair as fast as they GROW it.

Almost every black female in America, regardless to age or socioeconomic status, is experiencing some type of Hair CARE dilemma. The problems range from minor to extreme forms of damage breakage and hair loss. It is my mission and my passion to provide real solutions to these very real problems.

ShamBOOsie's Hair Wellness Approach to Hair GROWTH is a Real Solution Hair CARE Concept that was created to **Solve the 250-Year-Old-Hair-GROWTH Mystery!** What this book teaches will work to get your hair to GROW and Keep it GROWING and teach you Hair CARE. This incredible error-free System is the result of many years of research and hands-on testing. Finally there is a collection of products that effectively solve the myriad Hair-GROWTH difficulties that are unique to Black Hair and Women of Color.

We Didn't Reinvent the Wheel

With more than thirty years of experience in the beauty business, I have been able to pinpoint the major areas of concern for your hair. We didn't reinvent the wheel; we simply made the wheel work as it is supposed to. The trouble areas have been isolated and will be revealed to you. You will learn why you are experiencing so many

Beautiful Black Hair

problems with your hair and how to fix them. You will learn to identify the products that are damaging to your hair.

Please Accept My Apology

My name is ShamBOOsie. As an Industry Consultant and a Hair CARE Professional, please allow me to apologize for the emotional pain and suffering you have experienced because of the frustration of rapid and extreme hair loss, difficulties in managing your hair and your children's hair, and a market inundated with inferior Hair CARE products that have possibly caused more problems than they have solved.

Too many of us have taken you for granted. This will never happen with **Shamboosie's Hair Wellness Approach to Hair Growth** because we have had a watchful eye on you and your hair for years. We are completely aware of your many hair problems, and we are determined to solve them. We hear your silent plea for help. We know what your needs are even when you don't, and it is our mission to fulfill those needs, if possible.

Carry your own shampoo and conditioner with you to the Salon because it's the one way to make sure your Hairdresser is always using the best Conditioner and Shampoo. The hair salon will not always use a **High-End Conditioner and Shampoo or Hairdressing!** You MUST make sure to always buy and use **Humectress Moisturizing Conditioner and Therappe Shampoo from Nexxus Products, and Crème Press Hairdressing and a regular hold Styling Stray from Dudley's Products.**

ShamBOOsie's Methodology delivers for you.

Chapter 1

ShamBOOsie's 24 Month-Hair-Growth Timetable

A Hair Wellness Approach to Hair Growth

An Intensive Formula that really works; **The 24 Month-Growth Timetable** is designed especially for women who have been combing a Chemical No-Lye Relaxer through their hair or those who have had their hair chemically relaxed with any Relaxer. In order to turn the condition of your hair around, the first and most important step is to get complete control of the extreme dryness. You must totally reverse the extreme dryness and maintain absolute control over the dryness. I want to make absolutely sure you understand!

The hair has to go through a complete metamorphosis from extreme dryness to extreme softness before the healing and restoration process can begin. This is only possible if you follow the plan exactly and use only the recommended products as stated in the plan. **Reverse the dryness, and stop the breakage!** There are changes you can make to advance the plan. The process can be done every two days or every three days, which will bring about the change from dryness to softness much quicker. The dryness hasn't gone away, but it's under control.

First Make the Commitment

A serious commitment is required in order to achieve success with *The 24 Month- Growth Timetable.* It can work for you; however, you must promise to never comb another No-Lye Relaxer Kit through your hair as long as you live and use only the quality conditioners and shampoos your hair deserves. If your hair is chemical free, by which I mean you don't use permanent hair color either, this Growth Timetable will work even better. *The 24 Month-Growth Timetable* will help you reach your goal of maximum hair growth.

The expected new growth is approximately one-quarter to one-half inch per month. This is in addition to most of the hair you already have; you can expect to have the hair trimmed or cut along the way. This process will only work if you follow the program and instructions **EXACTLY and** use **only** the products and schedule the system requires. The product is the key and the most important aspect of the plan! You must NOT **Substitute or Eliminate ANYTHING** from this program. If you do, the extreme dryness and excessive hair breakage will return. TEST ME and prove me wrong. I am positive the System will work exceptionally well. *This is impossible with the products you may have on hand and about 98 percent of the CHEAP products made for use on Black Hair.* Those products are not designed to perform as well.

The Magic Formula

It is best to start with a *Conditioning Program. First "Reverse the Dryness and STOP the Breakage!"* The *Cuticle Layer* is much stronger than the fiber inside of each hair strand. In fact, the *Cuticle Layer* protects the inside like the eggshell protects an egg or your skin protects your insides. The use of No-Lye Relaxers has caused all three layers of your hair to act and feel like a single layer and become brutally DRY, hard, and resistant.

The ONLY way to change this is with a series of four to six conditioning applications done every three to four days. The closer together you can administer these conditioning applications, the quicker the process will reverse the extreme dryness and render the hair "cottony soft." Reversing the dryness is the most important part of *The 24 Month- Growth Timetable. Reverse the Dryness and, STOPS the Breakage!*

After each application, give the hair a day or two to absorb the moisture from the application. Each day the hair will absorb more and more of the moisture from the conditioners and the hairdressing, and the hair will become softer and softer. No single application of the moisture will be enough to fill the strands of your hair with what it needs to remain soft continuously. It will require several applications of three conditioners.

The needed moisture is applied in three forms: the *Moisturizing Shampoo, Concentrated Moisturizing Conditioner,* and the *Crème Press Hairdressing,* which is applied lightly, each day after the hair is blown dry and before styling. There is a fourth *Protein Conditioner* that will come into play four to six months down the road, after the dryness and the breakage have been brought under control. The *Protein Conditioner* is the strengthener and can ONLY be applied to the hair when it is soft. This conditioner must be able to penetrate the hair shaft and strengthen from the inside out, which is only possible when the hair is soft.

Please Note: It is not possible to stop your breakage, get your hair to grow, or to ever have healthier hair until the dryness is brought

17

completely under control. This takes priority over every other phase of *The 24 Month-Growth Timetable*. Remember this is ONLY **"the Magic Formula"** that makes real hair growth possible. These Moisturizing Conditioners are especially designed for maximum effectiveness in restoring and maintaining the exact moisture balance within the hair shaft. The System is by no means restricted only to chemically relaxed hair. **"The Magic Formula"** really works, and when used as directed, it will leave every texture of hair (relaxed, natural, or otherwise), smoother, silkier, softer, and more flexible so that the hair will bend rather than pop and break.

If you were to come to me today for service, the first thing I would do is prepare your hair for the application of a **Conditioning LYE Relaxer**. This **Conditioning LYE Relaxer** is the best chemical relaxer ever made for use on your hair. If you are now using a Lye Relaxer but once used a No-Lye Relaxer, the effects of the No-Lye Chemical are still in the hair. It will cause your hair to be dry occasionally. Eventually that hair will be eliminated. So if you are using a **No-Lye Relaxer, STOP** using it now and promise never to use it again. **The No-Lye Relaxer IS NOT a part of this program!**

I call the **No-Lye Relaxer** a **"Dehydrating Monster"** because it is the reason the hair is so dry that it has been impossible to reverse. This dryness is why your hair is breaking at such an alarming rate. The No-Lye Relaxer is also the most destructive product ever created for use on hair. Spread the word!

The Application Process
Conditioners in general are not designed to be effective after more than three days with only one application. To make them work, you need to build a foundation of conditioner so that it will last longer and will always remain effective. Therefore, conditioning every three

to four days will allow the conditioner to build a solid layer of protection on the cuticle layer of every strand of your hair. This allows it to soften and strengthen the inside. With the use of superior products, the hair will become softer, stronger, healthier, and more resilient with each application. I recommend reading the chapter on conditioners two to three times to get a complete understanding of how conditioners work. Nothing you do for your hair could be more important.

If it is about time to get your new growth relaxed, go ahead and begin *The 24 Month-Growth Timetable* by shampooing and conditioning the hair three times, once every two days or three times in six days. Then WAIT three more full days before getting the hair relaxed. This will prepare your hair for the first chemical application. After the **New Growth Relaxer,** proceed with the process for reversing the dryness. Don't Self-Apply any chemicals, please!

After the New Growth Relaxer or Retouch:
The following process MUST take place every three or four days for six times or until the hair is very soft to the touch. Then shampoo and condition your hair at least once a week and always on the same day. If the hair starts to feel dry again, do two to three treatments closer together. This program will not work if you are not consistent. You cannot just shampoo and condition your hair whenever you have the time. Nor can you skip a week or two and make it work. If your goal is to GROW beautiful healthy hair, it will require a sincere degree of dedication and diligence on your part.

If the objective is to make your severely damaged hair healthy again--*this is not possible.* However, we can improve on the health of your hair. Our objective is to help you keep the hair you have in place until we can help you GROW new hair to replace the damaged hair.

19

Protect the hair by applying a thin coat of *Crème Press Hairdressing* to every strand before hot curling or using a flat iron. (This will take a while, so take your time and do it right). The application of the *Crème Press Hairdressing* is the most important stage of the care process.

Reverse the Dryness, and STOP the Breakage!

Application Method (Crème Press): wait until the hair is dry to apply *Crème Press Hairdressing*. Take a dime-size portion and rub it between the palms of your hands. Rub the hands together rapidly to create friction and heat. This will cause the hairdressing to become very thin. Cover your hands and between the fingers with the hairdressing, so that application is easier. It only takes a very thin, very light coat of the product on each strand to work. You can always apply more where and when needed, even throughout the day. Use a very light, gentle touch during the application. Apply *Crème Press Hairdressing* every day so that the hair NEVER becomes dry.

This is Very Important!

Reverse the dryness, and STOP the breakage! The application of **"Dime-Size Portions"** is necessary to control the amount of the hairdressing you are applying. You are not using *Crème Press Hairdressing* for sheen alone.

Moisture in the hair simply means softness, not wetness. The moisture content of *Crème Press Hairdressing* actually repels heavy moisture. It is effective on different types of moisture that the hair does not need like the moisture in the air on a rainy day and even sweat. When applied lightly to every strand of hair, *Crème Press Hairdressing* seeps into the cortex, then returns to coat the cuticle layer with an amazingly brilliant, beautiful sheen not *shine*, and it softens the hair. The softness increases with each application, and the hair remains soft all day, then all week long. **You may also add some** *Styling Spray,* **if needed, and style as usual.**

The surface of the hair shaft is very similar in appearance to the scales of a fish—overlapping, tight, shiny, and slippery when the hair is healthy and wet. The hair fiber has a translucent protein outer layer consisting of seven to twelve cuticle cell structures; when they are very badly damaged, the hair can never be returned to its original healthy state. The superior conditioners contained in this System are designed to help keep the hair, even in poor condition, as healthy as possible.

- *The Shampoo Treatment* is formulated for stressed or chemically processed hair. It will soften and strengthen the hair as it improves elasticity and pliability, and replenishes essential softening properties. It is the perfect shampoo to work hand in hand with the conditioner.
- *The Concentrated Moisturizing Conditioner* will return more of the needed moisture to the hair with each application. It will intensify and accelerate the softening process and strengthen the hair as it improves elasticity, pliability and replenishes essential softening properties.

Always allow the conditioner to remain on the hair, under a plastic cap and under a warm dryer for fifteen to twenty minutes. Rinse well.

- *Crème Press Hairdressing from Dudley's Products.* Once the hair is blown dry, this product is to be applied in dime-size portions only. Use as much as needed to cover all of the hair but in dime-size portions. Every strand of the hair MUST receive the application. Take a dime-size portion of *Crème Press Hairdressing* and rub it between the palms of your hands until it is very thin.

21

If you press the palms together and rub them together really fast, it will create a little heat, which will cause the cream to become very soft and thin. Ensure that the crème is spread between the fingers also. Then with the fingers spread apart, apply the product with a "VERY LIGHT TOUCH." It will take some time to cover all the hair, but it is very important to do so.

Crème Press Hairdressing **is the most important of all** the products and the best there is for dry hair. It must be applied daily in the same way to keep the hair soft. *Crème Press Hairdressing* will relieve your hair of ALL the dryness. You may hot curl daily and safely with an electric iron if you use *Crème Press Hairdressing* to protect the hair from the heat. It will also keep the hair nice and soft. Styling spray will help the curls to hold longer. When you spray on the *Styling Spray* comb through the hair and allow the hair to dry completely, add a smidgen of *Crème Press* to each section as you curl the hair.

The Proper Relaxer for the New Growth Relaxer

- This *24 Month Growth Timetable* will begin with your relaxer retouch.
- **DO NOT APPLY YOUR OWN RELAXER!** I seriously recommend a Salon Professional perform the chemical service. However, if this chemical service is to be done at home, remember it takes two people to perform this service—the one receiving the service and the other applying the chemical.
- Have the hair cut or trimmed as needed. Split ends are the worst kind of breakage. If length is what you are trying to accomplish, it is important to tell your stylist to trim only what is needed to remove the split ends, which is usually about one-quarter inch, in most cases. Stay clear of style cuts and ask to be shown how much will be trimmed beforehand.

- Apply setting lotion every time before blow-drying the hair. This will soften the cuticle layer and make the hair easier to detangle when wet.
- Visit the salon every four weeks to have the hair shampooed, conditioned, and set to give the hair a rest from hot curling. This will tie in with the conditioning treatment to soften and strengthen the hair.
- You may consider alternating hot curling and roller setting the hair every other week. You will find it to be much better for your hair. The *Crème Press Hairdressing* will compensate for ALL the dryness regardless of what is causing it. Never hot curl or flat iron the hair without it. Any time you can get away from hot curling and blow-drying it will be better for your hair. Always apply *Crème Press Hairdressing.*

This is NOT a method for making your damaged hair healthy again— that is impossible. I will teach you how to care for your hair, and I will teach the things that will *prevent* damage and keep the hair strong— the real secrets to real growth. *Preventive hair care maintenance* lets you do what is necessary to avoid the problems before they begin. Yes, you can really do a lot of things that will give you longer hair. All it takes is learning how. You can trust me to show you how to properly care for your hair and to give you the necessary tools that will work. This is what *Shamboosie's Hair Wellness Approach to Hair Growth* is all about—Discovering the Secrets of Growing Longer Healthier Hair.

Getting your hair to Grow is not the problem—your hair is growing just fine. *Keeping the hair you grow is the problem.* Every six, seven, or eight weeks you are retouching your **newly grown hair.** So **Keeping the NEW GROWTH in place is the real secret to GROWING YOUR HAIR.** It amazes me how simple it is to grow and maintain a very healthy beautiful head of hair.

Everything that you achieve in life requires some work. If you are willing to do the work, it is possible to **GROW** your hair as **LONG** as you want and keep it **HEALTHY**. It doesn't matter whether you chemically relax your hair or wear it natural. The important thing is to condition it well and keep it as healthy as possible. I will show you what to do when your hair is healthy AGAIN, and growing.

The Areas of Concentration
- Stopping the Breakage, undoing the extreme dryness, and making your hair softer and stronger all in ONE STEP.
- Hair Breakage from lack of proper care
- Hair color and No-Lye Relaxer, the most difficult hair to work with
- Hair color and Lye-Relaxer
- The right types of Relaxers to use
- The Right type Hair coloring to use
- Removing the yellow for gray hair
- Natural Hair and Hair color
- Natural Hair
- Caring for Baby's Hair
- Caring for The Curl
- The Curl and Breakage: the Switch to Relaxer
- The Curl and Breakage: Hair color
- How to Stop Breakage: The Curl

A superior Protein Conditioner or Hair Rebuilder is the best conditioner for this texture of hair. The process of application is most important when there is color and relaxer in your hair. The *Protein Conditioner* with *this system* was created to handle this type of hair situation. The objective is to keep the cuticle layer as tough and as strong as possible. Allowing the hair to go without the conditioners it needs, will leave the hair to "fend for itself." Once the cuticle layer of the hair erodes, there is no way to reverse the damage. For coloring from this point on, use only a permanent hair color formulated **without** ammonia. Both chemical services (relaxer and hair color) MUST be handled a Salon Professional.

Silver, Gray, or White Hair: The type of shampoo is the only thing that changes when there is a problem with *yellowing stains* in silver, gray, or white hair. The yellowing is very natural, but it must not be allowed to linger. Removing the yellow must be done immediately every time you see it, and the sooner the better. The yellow becomes more difficult to remove the longer it is allowed to remain on the hair. There are special shampoos for this problem; however, the conditioning process remains the same.

Your Hair and Sports-Related Lifestyles: Many women exercise daily. Whatever time of the day your exercise program takes place, it creates a specific issue of concern regarding the hair because when you exercise you sweat. Therefore, the hair has to be shampooed and conditioned each day. This is quite a bit of work when the hair is chemically relaxed. The concept called **"The Magic Formula"** goes hand-in-hand with **The 24 Month Timetable.** The "magic" takes place with the application of the **Crème Press Hairdressing.** This is the product that will keep your hair soft on a daily basis, which is the secret to getting you through the next twenty-four months. At the end of the twenty-four months it should be "smooth sailing." You will be amazed to see your hair truly healthy, and keeping is healthy will also be easier.

The 24 Month-Hair-GROWTH Timetable - Possibly six inches in a year, twelve in two years, plus what you have already. Hair Growth is about the perfect CONDITIONERS and regular application. Follow the plan, trust this BOOK, trust Product, and by all means trust ShamBOOsie.

Chapter 2

You Must SHAMPOO and CONDITION Your Hair!

As a black woman, when you Chemically Relax your hair, you want hair GROWTH and beautiful, healthy hair; beautiful curls, and long, flowing shiny hair is what you want most for yourself and your daughters. A regimen of Quality Conditioners, Shampoos, and an amazing Hairdressing are all a part of the needed package. It is impossible to keep your hair healthy and GROWING as it should if you use low-end, poor quality Hair Care Conditioners and Shampoos. This is especially true of Chemical Relaxers.

When I first got in the business of Styling Hair, I went through the required 1,800 hours and started working in a local salon. I was scared to death of just about everything. The first time I Chemically Relaxed someone's hair, I went into the supply room alone, and I actually prayed, Oh God please don't let me do anything to damage this Woman's hair and please don't let me burn her scalp! Then I returned to my styling chair and did the Chemical Application. I can promise you that it didn't get any easier for me for four or five years, and every time, I prayed that same prayer. I couldn't understand a simple comb-out of a roller set, so I would my Clients to comb-out their own hair.

Beautiful Black Hair

I added this section to the book so that you would understand what is necessary if you are ever going to Master the Art of styling, managing, Chemically Relaxing, and keeping your hair as beautifully curled as you desire it to be. Caring for your hair and keeping it healthy so that it will have a natural sheen, movement, and bounce is extremely easy for anyone to do. What is very difficult about managing Black Hair is doing everything the correct way, especially with regard to the use of No-Lye Relaxer. If you believe that the poor quality maintenance hair care products you have been using will ever work for you—they won't..

Substandard Hair Products of any kind (no matter what type of product) will cause you to lose every inch of your hair. This is exactly what has been happening to your hair. You Combed the Chemical No-Lye Relaxer Kit through your hair and (perhaps your daughter's hair), and immediately you started having serious Hair Care problems. Your hair became extraordinarily DRY, hard, and began to pop and break. You did things the wrong way, used the wrong method of application and the incorrect formula of Chemical Hair Relaxer. Then you self-applied the Chemical, which is the worst possible thing you could ever do to your own hair. Along with using the wrong type of Chemicals, you also applied what you assumed were Conditioner and Shampoo products that would help your hair. Yet instead of beautiful, healthy hair, you have had nothing but one problem after another, and you can't seem to get it to GROW. Most black women use all of the wrong types of Hairdressing, Oils, Gels, and even styling sprays. When you couple all of this with NOT knowing EXACTLY what you are doing with every aspect of every situation with your hair, and with every product, in the end you have dry, damaged hair for yourself and your daughters. A regimen of Quality Conditioners, Shampoos, and an amazing Hairdressing is what will change everything for your hair and your family's hair.

Everything that is applied to your hair must do some good thing for your hair such as Soften, Strengthen the Cuticle Layer, or to help your hair GROW and be as beautiful as you would like it to be. It really is that simple!

Everything Must Change

You must Shampoo and especially Condition your hair on a regular basis—there is no way to get around the needs of the hair. There is no way to have and GROW shoulder length or longer hair without using Conditioners. I cannot emphasize enough that it is essential that you use the right products because it's not the process of shampooing and conditioning that will give you beautiful hair. The products you use MUST be up to par! The scale MUST forever be balanced. If the health of your hair on a scale of 1 to 10 is 7, and you were to change the texture or the condition of your hair, say to the level 5, the scale must be balanced, every time. Only the use of a quality conditioner will do this and bring the condition of your hair back to level 7. You need to understand why typical Hair Conditioners will never work for your hair, even if they are High-End Products. You must use the correct products each and every time.

Black hair must often be Chemically Relaxed, using a very harsh chemical. Often the chemical black women elect to use is the most devastating and destructive type—the NO-LYE Relaxer Kit, which is NOT a Relaxer and does NOT relax hair! As you know, once the hair is relaxed, you must continue to Chemically Relax the hair. The Chemical Relaxer Application itself is a time-sensitive Application and must take place every two months or six times a year. The NO-LYE Relaxer causes extreme dryness and a host of other problems. The consistent use of a chemical relaxer and the extreme dryness it causes are such a part of your life that proper conditioning is essential, but most High-End Conditioning Products were not

29

Beautiful Black Hair

formulated to deal with your hair issues. No products were, and this is the main reason nothing is working. The products you need must be meticulously selected for their unique, EXACT, and special composition, in addition to being High-End Hair Care Products.

This has very little to do with name brands. Rather, it has to do with formulation, the quality of raw materials used to make the product, concentrated levels of humectants (softening properties) that attract and hold moisture into the hair, keratin protein that contains all nineteen amino acids found in the hair to strengthen it, polymers to improve the Cuticle, acidifiers that carry a pH of 2.5-3.5, and other protectors and safeguards. No one has ever made true conditioners for black hair because it not about skin color, it's about HAIR. This means there are great HAIR products that will work for your hair. I have done the research to discover them for you.

The scale between your chemical use and sustaining quality and strength of your hair MUST be balanced. Only High-End Hair Conditioner and Shampoo will do the job. The use of the perfect conditioners and shampoos is the only way to balance this scale. Every time you use a chemical relaxer or Permanent Hair Color on your hair, it takes a lot out of the hair that it needs to thrive and survive. The concentrated levels of humectants (MOISTURIZERS and Softeners), keratin protein, acidifiers, and other protectors must be restored following the application of every chemical process. Even if no chemicals are involved, the hair will still lose the properties and nourishment it needs to survive.

The struggle and expense of managing kinky hair is enormous because you will not learn what you need to know and STOP doing things to your hair that send everything into a tailspin! LEARN! You have gotten your hair into a state that it is even a lot for me to manage, and I am a thirty-four-year veteran of the business. But there is a way to minimize the cost and the difficulty of handling your hair. It will take time to GROW your hair to shoulder length, but once we get the hair to that point, it will become much easier to manage.

Today black women wear their hair much the same way as other women—in as many different ways as there are black women. It will be the most difficult to manage while the hair is GROWING from three to eight inches. When the hair is short and GROWING from three to eight inches, women of color will have to really put in some work because once the hair is Chemically Relaxed it removes the hair's ability to hold a curl. This means a black woman has to hot curl, wrap, roll, or flat iron the hair every day. The problem with that hair holding its curls has been solved with the use of a **Medium Hold Styling Spray** and **a little Crème Press Hairdressing.** From eight inches on, only a slight bend in the hair with a **ceramic flat iron and a little Crème Press Hairdressing,** and the hair will be fairly easy to manage. You are going to need some help to learn to care for your hair, and this book will provide the help and knowledge you need.

To relax your hair every six to eight weeks the cuticle and cortex layers of your hair have to be constantly strengthened and softened with a GREAT **Crème Press Hairdressing,** and a High-End Moisturizing Conditioner that contains a fortifier to make your hair resilient so that it will sustain six applications of Chemical LYE Relaxer a year. If you haven't been caring for your hair, that is shampooing and conditioning regularly, the hair will suffer the consequences. I know you dread the idea of shampooing and conditioning your hair, but it MUST be done or your hair won't hold curl like you need it to. Your hair has no shine, no body, feels unhealthy, and looks unhealthy because it *is* unhealthy. It's dry, sheds very badly and often, and you have just about had it with your hair.

So here's the reality, **you MUST shampoo and condition your hair eight to ten times between each application of chemical relaxer.** You MUST do three to four conditioning treatments before the first retouch and before starting this 24 Month Timetable. If you have just had a retouch, go right into the six to eight shampoos and conditioners that would normally be done over the next six to eight weeks. This may seem like a lot, but consider that your hair hasn't been properly conditioned or relaxed correctly. So, you need to catch up.

To prepare for a marathon you MUST get your body in shape. Consider the application of chemically relaxing your hair as a "chemical marathon," and you must get the hair in shape and keep it in shape if you ever hope to keep it on your head. You MUST also apply the **Crème** Press Hairdressing lightly every day to keep the hair **soft to the touch** and protect it from the heat of hot irons. The **Crème** Press Hairdressing is also one of your conditioners.

Cowashing

Like the better idea of **Prewashing, cow**ashing is a new concept finding its way all over the business. There's a MYTH that it's possible to wash your hair too often that has been passed around by black women for many years. It's as if some Little Lady Genie is going from generation to generation among black women. Nothing could be further from the truth! It is impossible to Shampoos and Condition too often.

To compensate for stripping your hair of all its OILS, nurturing properties, some Lady of Hair Wisdom has come up with a concept she called *cowashing*. It means to wash the hair in between your shampoos and CONDITIONERS with a conditioner. However, that's like mixing the dirt and dirty oils in your hair with the wonderful, expensive Conditioners that I recommend in this book. Well, there is no such thing as washing with a conditioner because a conditioner doesn't remove OILS and dirt from the hair. However, the idea of cowashing is better than allowing your hair to go for one of two weeks without a good Shampoo and a Conditioner.

You will get the most from your Conditioners if the hair is clean. The natural pore in each hair strand, which is between or beneath the Cuticle Layer, will be free of DIRTY OILS that clog the hair and prevent the wonderful nurturing properties from performing as well to soften, strengthen, and protect your hair. Cowashing is all right as long as you clean your hair first. Shampoo and Conditioner go together like a horse and carriage. You can't have one without the other—ever! Shampoo first, then condition.

The more you shampoo and condition your hair, using High-End Conditioning and Shampooing Products, the SOFTER, STRONGER, HEALTHIER, and LONGER your hair will become. GROWTH! It's not about what you remove from your hair when shampooing; it's about what you put back into your hair when conditioning. It's about the type of Shampoos and Conditioners you are using and the type of Conditioning Hairdressing you apply after the hair is blown dry and before using a flat iron or a curling iron. The Hairdressing must be **Crème Press** from Dudley's Products.

For the "Scalp Massage Therapy Session" **ShamBOOsie** uses ONLY two High-End Products: **Therappe Shampoo and Humectress Concentrated Moisturizing Conditioner from Nexxus Products.** As mentioned above, the Hairdressing must be **Crème Press** from Dudley's Products.

Black women are collectively spending $9 billion a year on hair products and related items. Eight out of ten black females are losing so much hair that they are wearing false hair or have NO hair due to a lack of knowledge, the use of low quality conditioners, and a lack of commitment to a healthy hair care routine. Over 98 percent of this $9 billion, which is seven times as much as white women spend on much more expensive hair Conditioners and Shampoos, is going into the bank accounts of Beauty Giants like L'Oreal Paris and Revlon. You should also know that L'Oreal Paris owns, formulates, packages, and sells most black brands of Chemical No-LYE Relaxer Kits and the majority of the substandard shampoos, conditioners, and cheap oils. Since L'Oreal makes both High- and Low-End black and white Hair Care Products. When selecting your Conditioners and Shampoos, choose White Hair Care Conditioners and Shampoos like Humectress Moisturizing Conditioner, Therappe Shampoo, and **Crème Press Hairdressing** from Dudley's Products.

You MUST Do the SHAMPOOS and CONDITIONERS every four or five days and there is no way your hair will ever do well without the Conditioners.

- You cannot allow your hair to wait until you feel like doing it.
- You cannot avoid the treatments as you may remember there is a treatment with every conditioner in this plan.
- You cannot allow the price of products you will need to deter you from using the higher quality Conditioner and Shampoo. Do whatever you have to do to get the products you need to properly care for your hair; you will save money—a lot of money—over time, and your hair will flourish.
- You cannot allow the difficulty of styling the hair to discourage you from shampooing and conditioning your hair on schedule.
- Do not let your "party time" or any other distraction stop you from putting your hair on the "front burner" for a change. Many

women want lovely, longer hair but don't want to do what it takes to get it.

- You cannot service your hair every other week, every three weeks, once a month, or twice a year and expect the hair "to agree." Your hair will fall right off your head.

- You cannot continue to use so-called, **"Black Hair Products"** or products with the face of a black woman on the label. Stop taking so many chances with your hair! These products are inadequate, and will not work. When you select Conditioners and Shampoos choose ONLY **white hair products!** Remember, a white Manufacturer makes BOTH.

- A leave-in conditioner, mayonnaise, homemade concoctions, facial soap, an all-in-one shampoo and conditioner, or dishwashing detergent are simply not good enough. *The proper shampoo is as important as the proper conditioners.*

- You cannot trade your idea of the right products for the products ShamBOOsie recommends in this book and expect to make it work.

- Perhaps you have told yourself, "I know why my hair won't GROW—I shampoo too often. I heard you shouldn't shampoo the hair often because it will dry out the hair and scalp." As I mentioned earlier, this is a myth.

If your life is too busy to care for your hair, your hair will become too weak for you to look good. If you want it to look good and GROW, do the treatments. You must not allow anything to interfere with doing the shampoos and especially the conditioner because it is "a matter of life and death" for your hair. Make as many excuses as you want. The hair will not wait for you to make a decision to take care of it. It will fall right off your head if you don't! Take the time to put together a schedule for servicing your hair. Then commit to sticking to the schedule.

Beautiful Black Hair

You Get by with a Little Help from Your Friends

If you don't do anything else to your hair, please allow *the conditioning* to take place. You MUST do the shampoos and conditioners every four to five days to protect and preserve your hair. You must find someone to help you with your hair, which is why I have created **the Shampoo and Conditioner Massage Therapy Session!**

If your hair is in trouble, getting the hair of your dreams will require a lot of work for a very short period of time, and you will need a little help from a friend. You have to shampoo and condition the hair anyway, so you might as well do it the right way. Do it so that you and your hair will benefit from it. That's where **the Shampoo and Conditioner Massage Therapy Session** comes in to play. Ladies, the idea is to teach *someone of your choice* (human, your man, or significant other) to help you take better care of your hair. Trade the service by doing your Brother, Daughter, Girlfriend, Mother, Relative, or Sister and have that person do your **Shampoo and Conditioner Massage Therapy Session!** The goal is to create an enjoyable *pampering* experience in the process of shampooing and conditioning your hair. Let the wonderful, thick products do all the work. Set aside the time so that it can be done properly.

Use your imagination…Don't be afraid to ask your man to help you but be sure he follows the instructions in this book. Create some ambiance with music and candles, and so on. Be sure to put on a touch of your favorite perfume, and then let the pampering begin. You'll love it and he'll love it and most importantly, your hair will love it! If your situation doesn't lend itself to such a scenario, then ask your sister or girlfriend or daughter to help you. The "helper" doesn't have to be a man, although the massage sessions would be a lot more fun. What's important is that you get help with the shampoo and conditioning process.

In my, **"Let's Talk Hair Seminars"** women will almost pass out when I tell them the hair will need to be shampooed and conditioned every three to four days, with specific hair care products, in order to reverse the uncommon dryness caused by the No-Lye Relaxer. They will come up with every excuse imaginable to get out of shampooing and conditioning the hair every three to four days for four to six weeks. But if they do it, their hair will GROW AND GROW AND GROW! It's the only way to make the hair as healthy as possible. Once the dryness and breakage is under control, you may cut back to shampooing and conditioning once every five, six or seven days.

A Shampooing and Conditioning Massage Therapy Session How the Scalp Massage Affects Your Hair and Scalp

A warm conditioner massage has many benefits, and it should be done at least once every three, four, or four days.

* It cleans your hair and scalp very well. It stimulates blood flow, which is always a good thing because it helps to feed hair follicles with the nourishment they can only get from your blood. You want your hair to have the best chance to GROW healthy and prevent hair loss.
* It is extremely relaxing, calming, and helps relieve muscle aches and headaches. Your hair will become healthier with each massage session and application of the conditioner. The more sessions the better; the conditioners will make your hair feel terrific no matter who helps you do it.
* The most obvious benefit is it helps protect your hair from the damaging effects of the chemicals, cheap products, and the environment.
* The hair MUST be shampoo and conditioned; there's no way to avoid it and keep the hair.

- Shampooing and conditioning helps soften the hair and keep it soft and more manageable.
- It helps increase blood circulation in the scalp and neck area. When the scalp is "tight" from stress, circulation and hair growth are impeded. This is why I recommend applying a light covering of Vitamin AD&E scalp oil from Dudley Products on the scalp. It will increase pliability (soften the scalp), making the scalp stretch and move freely as it should. It helps to relax the scalp.
- It strengthens hair follicles, and the roots of your hair. It promotes new hair GROWTH and nourishes the hair shaft.
- It replenishes and rejuvenates dry, damaged hair and helps prevent excessive brittleness and split ends.
- You will sleep a lot better.
- You get to create your very own *spa-like* retreat in your home.
- You will discover a feeling of total calm and relaxation.
- It will save you a lot of money on salon services and free up more money for you to purchase the High-End hair conditioners and shampoos you will need to restore your hair. You will never get the GROWTH you want with the products you are now using.
- The weave is not all it's cracked up to be, and sooner or later it will leave you completely bald. It is a way to ensure the hair will not GROW.
- I can easily teach you or someone else how to give the most wonderful, most romantic shampoo and conditioning massage therapy session that you have ever experienced (romance is optional).

When a man touches your hair or gets close to you, you want your hair to feel soft and smell really good. He will notice and love the way it feels when it's soft. The Shampoo and Conditioner is scented and smell so good he will place his face close to you hair so that he can experience that fragrance. That's the way your hair should feel and smell. This is not the case with many black women's hair, but it can be. You want your hair to GROW, be healthy, and be as lovely as possible not hard or stiff-looking like little needles. And you want all of the hair on your pretty little head to be **"Your own REAL hair."**

As a man and a Hairdresser, I notice everything about a woman—I mean everything. I notice a woman's face and all its features, her smile and whether it lights up her face. Without effort I will notice her eyes, their size and color, and I can see right into her heart. I notice the way she walks, talks, her laugh, her soft-spoken mannerisms, how she is dressed, her beauty, which is far more than what my eyes can see, her personality, and charm. I see those things that are *only* about her, and I see the things every man should notice about her. It's no wonder God created a black woman last. My wife will tell you that I always take notice of the way she smells, if she is wearing perfume, and I wonder if she selected it just for me? Of course, I will always notice a woman's hair, whether it's her own or not.

If the man in your life is sharp, he will notice your hair—how it smells and feels. He may or may not say it, but I can assure you he notices. High-End beauty Conditioner and Shampoo products cost more, but you always pay more for quality, and aren't you worth it? Let's face it, there is no way you can continue the way you are going with your hair. You need to ONLY use Shampoo and Conditioner that WORKS, and you need someone to help you care for your hair. If you wait too much longer, you could *run out of real hair* because of breakage. Wearing false hair costs 100 times more than it will cost to manage your real hair and GROW it past your shoulders.

You are going to need quite a few conditioning treatments to get things back on track and beyond with your hair. Each *massage therapy session* comes with a high-end conditioning treatment that is better for your hair than anything you will ever use. The hair becomes stronger, softer, and healthier with each treatment.

Finding someone that knows and really understands black hair is like trying to find a needle in a haystack. That's an old Southern saying I grew up with, which means it's next to impossible. Women from everywhere e-mail me asking if I know of a salon in their area with someone that understands their hair. I don't have that information, but the pair of hands to give a relaxing shampoo and conditioner massage may be standing right in front of you. I am speaking of a mother, sister, husband, male, or female friend who could help. If you had someone to help you manage your hair from time to time, perhaps you would commit to doing what is needed to restore your hair. Nearly every black woman you know has the very same challenges.

For the life of me, I have not been able to figure out how to put your hair in the hands of someone who loves your hair as much as I do. The most obvious person is someone who loves you or at least likes you. Every black female needs to shampoo and condition her hair every three, four, or five days with good product and the perfect product for black hair. This will not be a so-called **Black Hair Product;** in fact, I wouldn't use **a Black Hair Product (cheap)** for all the tea in China.

I think my wife may have come up with the perfect solution. Who do you know that loves your hair as much as I do or loves you very much? She could very easily be your best friend, and it would make sense to do one another's hair, since the hair MUST be shampooed, conditioned, and styled OFTEN! I am talking about giving a shampoo and conditioning treatment and an amazing scalp massage at the same time. In other words, do a massage often and allow the shampoo and conditioner to be the product you use.

Imagine how much more enjoyable, and even romantic, the scalp massage would be if your man cared enough to help you out from time to time. With my help, you could teach him how to do it; I believe it's possible he could easily learn to help you care for your hair. The conditioning therapy session would be perfect for *his hair also*. Put it to the test; ask him to let you give him a scalp massage and use shampoo and conditioner. It doesn't matter how long or short his hair is he will love it, even without the massage. A great shampoo feels entirely different when someone else's hands are massaging the scalp. Dial his number and invite him over.

It Feels Really Great!

When it's done the right way—ShamBOOsie's way—it will cause you to close both eyes and if he is saying something to you while he's doing it, you shouldn't hear a word he is saying. It happens with my clients all the time. So make sure he takes his time and does it right. My mother would say, **"You have to teach a man how to treat you."** So, teach him! And if he gets the hang of it, he will be a keeper—which I can promise you. The expression I see on my client's faces says, "Oh that feels truly fantabulous," which means *fantastic* and *fabulous* all rolled up in one!

My clients like long shampoos and even longer conditioning sessions. This is why I set aside plenty of time to really take good care of each client. It takes time to truly do a great job of pampering them, and they will always pay me handsomely in the end, plus give me a big tip. Even if you could convince him to shampoo and condition your hair now and then it would be well worthwhile.

Here's How to Get Him to Agree!

I want to teach you a way to create your own *Hair and Scalp Massage Spa Retreat* in your own bathroom. When you need your hair shampooed, or you have a salon appointment for the end of next week, ask

41

him to shampoo and condition your hair. Have him follow the special instructions to the letter. It will quickly become a time for pampering, indulgence, and an opportunity for some real quality time with each other. Isn't this a wonderful idea? It's an incredible way for him to show you just how much he loves you. Don't you agree?

My clients are very special to me, and I appreciate their business. I always want to make the salon experience a really relaxing time for them. I take my time and do it right every time with every client. When the shampoo and conditioning part of the service is handled with special attention to detail, it can be very enjoyable.

Put on the largest of his T-shirts that you can find. Things will probably get a bit messy the first time, and there is likely to be water everywhere. As a hairdresser, I know what I'm talking about. The only objective is to have your hair shampooed and conditioned on a regular basis. He won't *always* feel like doing it, but the times he does will help you and your hair tremendously. If this works and you know that it will, I can promise you that you will never again have to concern yourself with finding someone to shampoo your hair.

As a woman with a busy life style, you must provide yourself with special, quiet time just for you. Self-indulgence doesn't get better than this. You can be completely pampered with a hair and scalp massage therapy session tailored to suit your needs. In addition you can finish with a long, warm relaxing double-bubble bath for one or two to really unwind and literally let your hair down. It's a perfect antidote to the stresses and tensions of modern living!

Love is a wonderful experience, and I will tell you there isn't anything I wouldn't do for my wife to make her day a better day. Such indulgence is ideal for those of us who lead busy, stressful lives.

This can be a beautiful and emotional experience that can bring two people closer together.

Pampering of this kind is a love session and love sessions can always help. It's also a two-sided coin: after he finishes lovingly massaging your scalp, you can immediately return the favor. Many of my clients return to my chair because I make their visit to the salon so relaxing and so special each time. It is really simple and easy to do. I just treat each client like the lady she is.

If there is no special friend, husband, or significant other, simply remove him from the equation, but keep your evening of pampering indulgence. There will still be ways of making it a most wonderful evening to relax, unwind, and immerse yourself in a well-deserved moment of self-indulgence. This pleasurable indulgence would be a special gift just for you and just because!

Now Let's Build a Spa in Your Place

There are two places in the home where there is running water and where a treatment could be done with a second person involved: over the sink in the kitchen or on your knees bending over the side of the bathtub, using a showerhead. The kitchen sink will normally have a hose with a sprayer, but one would have to be installed in the shower.

The bathroom can easily become a special place for total relaxation. It is the perfect place to revitalize, wind down, and just relax. The bathroom is normally a room occupied by a single person, but in the case of a massage therapy session, it must become a room for two. If your bathroom is small and there's not enough room, move to another area in your home. You mostly need the bathroom or kitchen for the water, but no water is needed during the *massage phase.* All that is on the hair during the scalp manipulation and massage is the conditioner.

You are going to need a few things to get set up. We are going to transform your shower and bathroom into a luxurious retreat, with a soothing and relaxing showerhead. It makes every shower a spa-like experience if you purchase the right one, so shop around! They don't cost that much, are easy to install, and it will be a one-time purchase.

The showerheads come with several personalized shower settings for individual comfort such as steady pulsating sprays, a turbopulse, powerful hyper massages, a pulsating, full soft-body spray, a center spray, and forceful concentrated spray. Sometimes the water moves with up to 2,800 pulses per minute. It all can be easily adjusted with an outside control dial. There are many different brands and types to choose from. Look for one with many settings and a way to start and stop the water, using the sprayer. Once you install it, the system can remain in place for the whole family to use. These showerheads come with a wall mount that allows you to use it like your regular shower.

These showerhead Massages are amazing. When you are not having your hair and scalp massaged, shampooed, and CONDITIONED with High-End products, you'll enjoy a long, hot, relaxing shower where you have the ability to move the water and place it where it's needed most, for example, in the middle of your back, neck, and across your shoulders. Now imagine that the water is moving just as you want it, with the temperature precisely to your liking. You can step straight from this magical interlude into your daily life, refreshed and renewed every day if you want. And your hair will be healthy, clean, and very well conditioned. And just imagine, your hair becomes easier to manage when it has GROWN to shoulder length or longer.

When you open your bottles of Nexxus Therappe Shampoo and Humectress or Keraphix Conditioners, take time to smell them. They will leave your hair smelling clean, fresh, and really nice. Imagine yourself totally embraced in a gentle stream of water cleansing your body, mind, spirit, and hair.

At this rate you may now find the time to shampoo and condition your hair as often as it needs to be in order to restore it. We are talking about three times in a ten-day period for the first month to six weeks, then every four to five days to give the hair the nourishment it needs. You could get used to this really fast with "a little help from your friend." (If you are wearing a weave, this therapy session will not work. False hair doesn't need conditioning.)

Practice Makes Perfect!
There are some things you have to teach a man to do. In this case it will be his learning to handle the massage therapy session. Never rush it! It will require a few practice sessions to get it right. Unless your man is a Hairdresser, talking him into conditioning your hair might not be so easy. In fact, he may hate the idea until you show him all the ways the two of you will benefit from the experience. You may want to find just the right atmosphere to suggest the idea to him.

The purpose is to get you a little help. He may even learn to help you dry the hair using a comb attachment on the end of a hair dryer. Just take it one step at a time, and remember there is always mother, sister, or girlfriend you can call on to give you a little help.

To make this really work, you need to answer a few questions for yourself that will help you do these massage sessions the right way so that you will have everything ready and in place, when and if he agrees to do this for you. These questions pertain *only* to the massage sessions between you and "someone special."

- **What should you wear?** As little as possible and never your good clothing. Wear something you don't mind getting wet like a shirt without a collar. You want to make as little mess as possible. Make sure bathrobes, slippers, and towels are provided for your and his use. You may also need a pair of earplugs to help keep the water out of your ears.
- **How long should you allow for this experience?** You will need approximately two hours. When no massage will take place, and the hair will only be shampooed and conditioned, it will only take about thirty minutes to complete.
- **So when does the activity take place?** As the woman and because this is more about you than him, you must decide; you hold all the cards. All he has to do is show up and get busy. There is a possibility of this happening at any time of the day, any day of the week, and all year round.
- **What is the minimum age is for the message therapy session?** As long as you are an old enough woman to alone with an adult male for two hours. If the hair is to only be shampooed and conditioned, age doesn't matter.
- **What about the weather?** Rainy and snowy days are simply wonderful for the scalp massage therapy session, but any day is a great day to do something special for your lady. Rainy and snowy weather could have a very positive effect on this experience.
- **Should you bring spectators?** Sorry, it's for his eyes only!
- **What else do I need to know?** Know that you are in complete control but make him believe he's the one in control.
- **What else will I need to round out the evening?** Now it's getting personal...to start the evening, put on some soft music, love songs, soft jazz, perhaps Baby Face or Luther Vandross. You are

about to spend some real quality time feeling beautiful and special. And your hair and scalp will love every minute of it. If the phone should ring, let the answering machine pick up the call. Leave the message that you're busy being pampered and ask callers to leave a message.

- **What else?** Light a few scented candles and place them conspicuously around the room. Place a lamp with a low-wattage red bulb in the room. It has a way of quieting and softening the room. Ambience helps set the perfect mood. Prepare some chocolate-covered strawberries, and your favorite wine or beverage. One or two bottles of a sweet wine, perhaps some **Beringer White Zinfandel from California (2005)** will do the trick. You will love it! Use your best wine glasses. Be picky with the glasses—they should be sexy and as lovely as you want to feel.

Be sure to include all you special perfumes, body oils, bubble bath, Shea butter, creams, and lotions. The minimum cancellation notice once the event is scheduled should be forty-eight hours. He better not think of canceling any time after that. I love to get gifts and give gifts. He should know that this is better than candy and flowers, but that candy and flowers would be appreciated anyway.

Lovely Smelling Fragrances—HINT, HINT!

A few Christmases back my wife and I traveled south for the holidays. I always manage to surprise her with a gift. Just before packing for the trip, I went to the mall to shop for my wife's gift. I never like this job, and I guess a lot men feel the same way. So I spent a couple of hours walking through the mall but not finding what I wanted to buy her. I came across a Bath and Beauty Store and went in to see what they had. I was in the store for about an hour, and picked out an enormous assortment of lotions, bath oils, creams, bubble bath,

47

special hand and facial soaps with Shea butter in them, and some *lovely smelling fragrances.* She loves this kind of stuff.

It took me so long to shop because I had to smell everything to see if I liked it. Then I had to find a way of carrying all with us on the trip without her knowing. I went to another store and bought a big box that was covered beautiful red silky quilted fabric. I packed all of the goodies into this pretty silk box. But there was still the problem of hiding it. I managed to get it into the house without her seeing it but didn't know I would be able to transport it.

When it was time to leave for the trip, I told my wife to start loading her things into the car, and that I would carry the heavy suitcases. She had packed a large suitcase for herself and while she was putting the smaller things in the car, I slipped the red silk box with all the goodies into her suitcase. I zipped her suitcase up and packed it into the car.

I didn't say a word about the gift the entire twelve-hour trip. When we reached our hotel room, I waited and waited for her to open her suitcase and discover the gift. It seemed like it took forever. I kept hinting and hinting, but I didn't want to give away the surprise. Finally, I started to unpack a few of my own things, and then she followed suit. I wish you could have seen the look on her face when she found the gift. I have to tell you, I got to enjoy all of the "goodies" and lovely smelling fragrances for many months to come.

Your Personal Pampering Getaway

Occasionally you can take the act on the road. Everyone likes to be pampered a little now and then. Where this wonderful indulging experience takes place will be up to you. Be creative. Whether the kitchen, the bathroom, the bedroom or all three, you have plenty of time to decide, but *you* must be the one to decide. It wouldn't hurt to take this act on the road once or twice a year to a lovely hotel. You may have to spend handsomely for the getaway, but aren't you worth it?

The hotel can be down the street, around the corner, just across town, or in another state. You work hard and deserve some "personal" time. A *shampoo and conditioner massage therapy session* is even better when you make it part of a weekend getaway. Use your imagination, be creative, and treat your hair in the process.

Remember that Moisture Means Softness

When your hair is dry, it isn't soft. Moisture in the hair simply means softness not oiliness or wetness; it's *in* the hair, not *on* the hair. This is the purpose of the Conditioning Lye Relaxer, Moisturizing Conditioner, Setting Lotion, Styling Spray (with the minimum alcohol content), most important thing and you can't ignore it. Moisture, (SOFTENESS) strength, and healthier hair are always your objective. Only when you do the shampoos and conditioners with the prescribed products is it possible to create moisture and strength your hair will always need. Healthy hair will not occur by any other means.

You MUST SHAMPOO and CONDITIONER Your Hair OFTEN

Why Use Only Quality Hair Care Conditioner and Shampoos?

Many of you will read this book and say to yourselves, "He keeps saying the same thing over and over." Isn't this what a good teacher is supposed to do? This is the most difficult thing to get people to comprehend. A thousand women will have a thousand different opinions about the type of product they use on their hair. They all can't be right. In fact, 97 percent of them are wrong. The products in this book are a selection from the cream of the crop. The most wonderful thing about these **Quality Hair Care Products** is they will do exceedingly above and beyond what you can imagine to keep your hair soft, beautiful, healthy, and *GROWING* strong. The more you use the right products the right way, the better the products will work, and the stronger, healthier, and more beautiful your hair will *GROW.* You can trust the products listed; each of them is excellent and so much better for your hair. My slogan is ShamBOOsie—the name you can trust! You can REALLY trust me because I care about your hair!

The Making of a Master Hair Designer

I teach women how to GROW Beautiful Healthy Hair. Growing healthier hair is all about doing everything correctly and includes using just the right **CONDITIONERS.** This doesn't mean just any jar of product with the word *CONDITIONER* written on its label. High quality conditioners are a part of the ingredients of every product on your list of needs. The types of raw materials used to make each product are of a Higher Quality with each product line. The very best really work like magic. But you must be meticulous with your selection!

Talking Heads

A newborn baby cannot speak a word, yet she has many ways to convey to her mother exactly how she feels about everything. The baby has a distinctly different cry or sound that she makes for different things she wants and needs. When I first became a father, I realized early on that new Moms quickly and instinctively learn to recognize the baby's every little whimper and to know exactly what each one means. The cry that says, "I don't feel so good because my diaper is really messy" is very different from the cry that conveys, "The new food you fed me today is some nasty stuff, and I don't want any more of it." But the most beautiful thing the newborn could say to her mother is **I love it when you take the time to care for me.** I love all of the nice things you rub on me that make my skin soft and smell good, and I can tell by the way you treat me that you really do love me because no body holds me the way you do.

Now what do you think your hair would say to you (if it could talk) if you treated it like a newborn baby? Would your hair know that you care? That really is the secret to GROWING longer, beautiful healthy hair. The way to determine what is best for your hair is simply to allow the hair to dictate. Allow your hair to "speak" for itself and listen closely to what it is trying to tell you. It will make all of the right decisions for itself. It knows more about itself than you or I will ever know. The hair will always make the best decisions for itself. Your job and mine is to allow the hair to teach us how best to treat it.

For more than thirty years, hair has taught me hundreds of things. I have made it a habit to listen very closely to what it says to me. Perhaps you didn't realize it, but your hair has been talking to you. Did you know that your hair loves to eat well, and almost as often as you do? It likes to be fed every day, but most people feed it whenever they get ready or not at all. If you could hear the "voice" of your hair, it would tell you:

1. The kinds of food it likes most.
2. That it likes only "the good stuff," and if you were really listening it would tell you, "Just because I am on a BLACK HEAD it doesn't mean I only like BLACK HAIR CARE PRODUCTS."
3. When it is hungry.
4. If it's too weak and just barely hanging on.
5. Whether or not it is a good idea to apply bleach or permanent hair color with ammonia in it.

6. When you have applied the right relaxer, and if it was applied correctly.

Now if your hair could really speak, it would probably say, "Please get to know me very well before you do something that I know will hurt or destroy me." **The way the hair actually "speaks" is visually.** We see the damage, the weird color, the lack of moisture, and we see when it has fallen out and is dying. When you look at your hair you can see that it is dry and lifeless, and has no sheen. Perhaps it pops and breaks, is puffs up, smells sour or dirty, or desperately needs to be shampooed and conditioned.

Most Important is the Toolbox – Here is What You Need

✓ Blow Dryer
✓ Comb Attachment – Willie Morrow
✓ A Champion #99 Shampoo Rake Comb
✓ Champion Tuff Comb 8" #28
✓ Twelve black tail combs (#263)
✓ If you can't find Champion combs, Ace Combs are a good replacement
✓ Cushion Brush and Vent Brush
Shop at Sally's Beauty Supply Stores.

When Working with Your Daughter's Hair

- After the hair has been shampooed and conditioned, spray on some setting lotion and allow it to sit on the hair for about five minutes.
- Towel dry the hair until it's damp. Always begin the drying process when the hair is damp, never completely dry. If the hair dries before you have the chance to use the blow dryer and comb attachment, have a spray bottle on hand. The stray nozzle on the bottle should spray a light mist, enough moisture to dampen the hair.

- Start by separating the hair into many small subsections. You can begin detangling the hair while separating it into the small sections.
- Begin combing at the ends, holding the hair firmly with one hand between the thumb and fingers to ease the pull on the hair. Comb from the ends of the hair toward the scalp, removing the tangles as you go along.
- Begin the drying process using your blow dryer with the comb attachment, and dry each subsection of hair completely. Make sure the hair is damp to the touch and dry the hair from damp to dry. Plait or braid the hair.
- Move to the next section, and repeat the procedure, until all of the hair is done. The plait, braid or hot press each section of the hair.
- Don't use heavy oils on her hair. The Crème Press will do very well.
- These techniques can be used until the child is seventeen years old or as long as the hair remains natural. The only difference when the hair is chemically relaxed is the detangling process. The hair will be easier to manage when it is chemically relaxed. It will be safe to chemically relax her hair anytime you decide as long as you care for the hair.
- Use ONLY the conditioners and shampoos mentioned in this book or throw the book away and do your own thing.

Is there a Way to Select the Right Salon?

This will be very hard to do nowadays because there are fewer of them, and the stylists in many black hair salons are deficient in their knowledge of your hair. When selecting a salon to take your daughter for her chemical relaxer, there are several things to look for in the stylist you select. Check to see if the stylist's hair is healthy. It the stylist is a woman, is she wearing a weave? Does the stylist have experience working with children's hair?

- Ask for referrals from other mothers, other women, and friends.
- Check out the salon; go and ask questions or ask your hairstylist for recommendations.
- Visit some of the different local salons in your area. Look around in other towns in your area.
- Look for stylists who have many clients that are children, and then go and observe their work.

You may have to search a bit, but you will find a stylist you can trust. Every stylist will not work well with kids. I have worked with many children over the years. Do your homework, ask around, look around, and don't just settle. When you have the chemical work done professionally, you will feel more comfortable doing the maintenance care for her hair and yours, at home. The stylist you select for your child can be entirely different from the person you have taking care of your hair.

Remember to stay away from cheap hair care products. When you locate the right salon for you and your child, it is a good idea to purchase your own conditioners and shampoos. Most black hair salons will not carry High-End conditioners and shampoos. Simply carry them with you and ask your stylist to use them on your hair and your daughter's hair. If the stylist doesn't allow clients to bring products into the salon, ask the stylist to purchase and use the products that you prefer. If the stylist doesn't go for that, the stylist can no longer complain about the products you bring with you. Whatever you do, don't allow anyone to talk you into believing the products I recommend are for white people's hair. The products recommended here are for anyone with hair, which is why they are called, HAIR CARE products and not skin care products. I recommend them because they work. When you find a stylist that you are comfortable with, stay with that stylist.

"Acoustic Soul" the CD from India Arie

I Must Recommend This Piece of Music. It is an older album of songs that every black woman and young girl should have. It is truly an expression of your natural beauty as a black woman and of the way you should really feel and think of yourself and who you really are. Then it will be a natural thing to pass it on to your daughters and the women you bring into this world. I personally think that the black woman is the most beautiful creature God has ever created.

Put Me and My Methodology to the Test

Little black girls wearing FALSE hair? That's Horrific! Little black girls across America and around the world are wearing some form of FALSE HAIR, weaves, braids, or extensions, and it is my mission to help them GROW their own beautiful healthy hair. I can't imagine a two-year-old little black girl wearing a weave, but I see it all the time, and it breaks my heart. It breaks their hearts, too.

Every time you get an extra ten or twenty dollars you can spend on products, go out and buy Keraphix Conditioner, Humectress Moisturizing Conditioner, and Therappe Shampoo. Buy the products in as large a size as you can afford and stock up on them. When applying, use small portions as to not waste the product. Use as much as you need to cover all the hair, but in small portions. Make a conscious effort to get the products you need. The products you need can be found in drugstores all over the country. So there is no excuse! Stop allowing the price of great hair care products to become a reason not to have and GROW lovely hair. **You can't do this without the Quality Hair Care Products—it's Impossible!**

A Hug and a Kiss from ShamBOOsie

Chapter 3

Instructions for: A Shampoo and Conditioning Scalp Massage Therapy

Be Pampered with an easy Scalp Massage. It's a Soothing, Relaxing, and Calming Twelve-Step Program. Every woman wants to feel special, and a little "touch therapy" for stress reduction is absolutely wonderful. I am completely bald and still find the scalp massage enjoyable. The massage therapy session will require three to four rinses, depending on the number of shampoos. The splash-free gentle rinsing action of the showerhead truly massages the scalp to rinse away the thick, creamy shampoo lather after the two to three shampoos, and after the fourth or fifth massage, one or two with only conditioner on the hair. The ones with the conditioner really feel the best. I know you can hardly wait for me to tell you how he should do the scalp massage.

The magic is in the pads of the fingers and just the right Love, Sensitivity, and amount of pressure. These instructions are for the person who will be doing the Conditioning therapy session. Everything begins at the wash station in the kitchen, over the bathtub, or in the shower using the five-foot hose and multi-action showerhead.

Begin your mind-relaxing ritual with a soothing foot soak. Buy a special soap or use whatever you enjoy. Allow the water to be as warm as possible but not hot. The foot soak can take place at the same time you are having the scalp massage therapy session. Or you may want to complete this part before moving on to the shampoo and conditioning session. The idea is to make an evening of it. Keep the conversation light and positive.

A third location is in the shower where you can do your own shampoo and conditioner. When the work is to be done in the kitchen or bathroom, place a large folded towel over the side of the counter or bathtub so you'll be comfortable when you lean over the tub or sink. You want to be as comfortable as possible no matter where it is done.

Whichever you choose, it will only be used when water is needed to wet the hair or remove soap and conditioner from the hair. Otherwise the actual massage can take place in a more comfortable setting like the living room, dining room, or bedroom.

Now massage the scalp for a minute or so while the hair is still dry. Do it slowly and gently, using only the cushiony pads of your fingers. Never use the fingernails no matter how good it feels, even if she asks you to. The nails will harm her scalp.

- Be sure the room is warm or cool enough for the both of you to be comfortable.
- Heat some water in a deep, small pot. I shouldn't be boiling because you'll place your bottles and jars of shampoo and conditioner in it to warm the products slightly.
- Seat her in a comfortable armless chair with a soft cushioned seat. Make sure she is very comfortable.

- To drape her for the shampoo therapy session, stand behind her, place a towel across her shoulders, cross the ends over each other under her chin, and then ask her to hold it in place.
- Place the cape over the towel around her neck and fasten it in the back so that the cape does not touch her skin, but is tight enough to keep her from getting wet. The shampoo cape must be made of plastic. A shampoo cape and can be purchased at beauty supply stores or drug stores for about $10.00. A good shampoo cape will save you from making a mess and make clean up much easier.
- Then place a second towel over the cape and secure it in front with a clip.
- Remove all hairpins and combs from the hair.
- Make sure she isn't wearing earrings or glasses. You don't want to get a finger caught in one of the earrings.
- Turn off the TV and turn on some music softly in the background.
- Gently comb through the hair with a large-tooth comb to remove any tangles. If you must talk, speak in a soft tone.
- Lean her gently forward over the sink and have her keep her eyes closed. She will need a small towel to dry her face along the way.
- Adjust the pressure and temperature of the water. Test it on the inside of your wrist. The water should be as warm as possible but not hot. She will let you know if it is too warm or too cool.
- Be sure to turn on the cold water first and keep it away from the hair and scalp until it's just the right temperature. Add hot water as needed. The water could change temperatures during the shampoo session so check it from time to time. Never allow the water to run cold and touch her scalp.
- Be very generous with the when applying the shampoo. You want the lather to be very thick like whipped cream. You can't imagine how completely tranquilizing it is.

Basic Scalp Manipulation Techniques

There are a few ways to effectively manipulate the scalp, but you want him to learn the most relaxing ways.

STEP 1: Wet the hair completely with warm water. Use a towel to remove only the water dripping from the hair but keep the hair wet enough to work in some shampoo to clean the hair. Apply a generous amount of shampoo and work it to a very thick, creamy lather. It should be thicker than whipped cream and almost as thick as whipped butter. You want to add the shampoo this way only the first time of each session.

STEP 2: With her hair wet and ready for the treatment, have the person receiving the scalp massage to sit in a comfortable chair. A kitchen or dining room chair is best. Add a small pillow if necessary. Make sure you can reach the back of her head comfortably with both hands. For the massage, spread your fingers and move slowly around the subject of the therapy session. This will enable you to work with her hair and scalp with only the balls of your fingers. The manipulations MUST be done sloooowly and in circles. Use different amounts of pressure. Don't forget to trim your fingernails before you begin, but NEVER use your fingernails because they will bruise the scalp.

The fascination about the therapy session is what happens with the rotation of the balls of his fingers. The amount of pressure used and the thick shampoo cream is what makes it feel so wonderful. The movements are slow and concentrated to intensify the process.

STEP 3: The massaging process actually begins with the conditioner and with you standing directly behind the subject. The fingers and thumbs will be moving in a circular motion, using small circles and larger circles other times. The pattern used is up to you; just go back and forth, and in circles all over the scalp. All of movements should be slow and there should be slight pressure on the scalp.

Place the balls of your fingers on each side of her head. Slide your hands firmly upward, spreading the fingers until they meet at the top of her head. Then repeat this motion several times. Move your thumbs in circles all over the back of the head and neck in a sliding and rotating movement. Just as in step one, rotate the fingers, and move the scalp around. Repeat several times.

STEP 4: Run some hot water into a container larger enough to hold the container of conditioner. Place the closed container of conditioner in the hot water and allow it to heat up. The conditioner should be warm but comfortable to the touch.

STEP 5: Using the balls of the fingers, apply the conditioner in small portions to all the hair; for this massage use a little more than normal. The full length of the hair should be covered with the conditioner. Remember that when the conditioner is High-End *the hair will receive a treatment with every application*. Otherwise none of this will make any sense.

STEP 6: Then, keep your fingers spread and use the balls of your fingers to move in a SLOW circular motion over the scalp. The movement must be deliberate and relaxing, and constant. Vigorous movements will enhance and speed up the circulation of the scalp.

STEP 7: Using the balls of the fingers of both hands, stroke the hairline around the forehead and toward the temple as if you were drawing four partings with your fingers between her brow and hairline.

61

STEP 8: While standing behind the subject, massage the forehead hairline along the front, side, and back of the head, making small slow circles with your fingers only for about three minutes. Then shift one step to your right or left and repeat the same circular motions for one or two minutes, and continue to shift your body one step to your right or left until you can't move any farther. Massage the scalp for two to three minutes. Next start moving one step in the opposite direction and massaging the scalp until you can't move any farther. Continue for twenty to thirty minutes.

Your hands should never stop massaging in circles and your hands should make a complete movement around the subject's head. Keep your hands on the scalp until the completion of the session or to add more conditioner. There is no hurry so take your time and move slowly, your hands and your body. Work your way toward the top of the head, as if drawing little circles with the balls or cushions of your fingers.

STEP 9: The scalp should be massaged every time the hair is shampooed and conditioned. Do not give up after a few treatments because the hair will give up if you do. Make it a habit to shampoo and condition your hair!

STEP 10: You can rinse and reapply the conditioner for a second scalp massage. Be sure to massage the entire scalp, gently in the temple area, down the front and back of the ears, back of the neck and everywhere there is hair on the head (every tiny little strand, no matter how short the hair is). This process should last at least twenty to thirty minutes, longer if you like.

Fold Take a towel that is large enough to wrap around the head, and soak it in hot water. Squeeze the water out and wrap the towel around the head after the massage is completed. This is a moisturizing conditioner and the moist heat will help infuse more conditioner and softness in the hair. After another twenty to thirty minutes, rinse the hair in the shower, using warm water and your multi-action massaging showerhead.

STEP 11: Use a smooth, slow, delicate stroke and apply more pressure now and then. Notice whether the scalp is moving, and then use smooth, slow, delicate strokes again. Some people's scalps will move more than others, but this is a good thing.

Chapter 4

Crème Press Hairdressing: Your Secret Weapon

It's the MAGIC in All ShamBOOsie Does for Beautiful Healthy Hair.

The secret is in the dressing. Your foremost challenge is to get control of what I call the Dehydrating Monster—the extreme dryness that comes from using the No-Lye Relaxer. Your Secret Weapon is **Crème Press Hairdressing** by Dudley. With Crème Press, this monster doesn't stand a chance.

The problems that make it impossible to get past the extreme dryness include the inability to keep moisture (SOFTNESS) in the hair after it has been blown dry and finding a way to keep the hair soft throughout the week. You must be able to keep your hair soft for as long as it takes to grow out of the damaged dry hair and into softer healthier hair, which will take about twenty-four months in most cases.

- **Crème Press**, when applied lightly to every strand of hair, seeps into the cortex, and then returns to coat the cuticle layer with an amazingly brilliant beautiful sheen not *shine*; it softens the hair. The softness increases with each additional application, and the hair remains soft all day, all week long.

- **Crème Press** actually repels heavy moisture, for example moisture in the air on a rainy day, and even sweat; those are two different kinds of moisture that the hair does not need.

- **Crème Press** will also repel and prevent the hair from drying out during the day, drying out from styling sprays that contain alcohol, and it stops the heat from hot irons from drying the hair out. So it's perfect for hot curling.

- **Crème Press** conditions the hair with every application. So it is important to use it in very small amounts. If a dime-size portion is too much, use half as much or an even smaller amount. With some hair, one dime-size portion may be all you need.

- **Crème Press** is the perfect crème for Pressing and Curling natural hair, which is what it was originally formulated to do.

- Considering all of the things **Crème Press Hairdressing** can do for your hair, its only job is to Dress the hair. It is a finishing sheen in crème form. You don't need anything else.

- **Crème Press Hairdressing** MUST be applied every day.

For many years I have been using **Crème Press Hairdressing,** and I've been aware of its incredible capabilities. I am never without it— no matter for whom I'm working. When I worked for various hair care companies, I would keep my **Crème Press** in secret containers and call it my "Magic Potion." I would never tell anyone what it was. I have never found any other product that performs as well. **Crème Press** is just that good!

Styling Spray:

There are hundreds of styling sprays on the market, and I have used many of them, although nothing else compares to **Styling Spray by**

Dudley. It is a very unique tool because you get to CONTROL its use. You decide how much hold you need with this styling spray. Other sprays come in separate cans for different intensities of hold. The alcohol content in **Styling Spray by Dudley** is minimal, so when used correctly, it will never dry the hair out.

If it does cause a bit of dryness, the unique moisturizing ingredients in **Crème Press Hairdressing** have the ability to cancel the dryness, leaving the hair with strong curls that will last and remain soft to the touch all day long. You can make the hair as hard as a brick or as soft as a baby's bottom. I have made curls hold for a week without the hair becoming hard to the touch. (I can't stand for the hair to be hard, and there is no reason why hair should ever be hard.)

Blow Dry and Hot Curl Every Day
Styling Spray used in conjunction with **Crème Press Hairdressing** becomes magic in your hands. You can hot curl and use both products every day without drying out the hair. These two products will give you **absolute control** over the way your hair holds curls, its shape, and style; plus you have **absolute control** over every aspect in the styling process.

In addition, **Crème Press Hairdressing and Styling Spray** conditions the hair with every application. That's a lot of positive performance from just two products in **the Hair Wellness Approach to Hair Growth.**

Crème Press Hairdressing is by far the best hairdressing ever created for use on black hair. **Crème Press** is designed to coat and protect the hair from the damaging effects of excessive thermal or blow-drying heat.

It works exceptionally well, and it is never oily. It improves the texture of relaxed hair by giving it a SOFT, SATINY, and SILKY look and feel. It is a moisturizing conditioner that strengthens, softens, and restores moisture in the hair shaft no matter how extreme the dryness is.

Because the softness **Crème Press** creates becomes even softer over time, daily use of this product keeps the hair soft, which helps to bring the breakage to a complete stop. There is no way to take control of the extremely dry hair without **Crème Press Hairdressing.** I have tried and tested many other oils and hairdressings searching for solutions over the years, and nothing worked until I used **Crème Press Hairdressing.**

Crème Press must be applied after the hair is blown dry and always before curling the hair. This hairdressing leaves the hair with incredible softness and sheen that lasts all-day and longer. After about twenty minutes, the hair takes on BEAUTIFUL, BRILLIANT SHEEN after using **Crème Press Hairdressing.** I have never used a product that was capable of doing what Crème Press does so well.

What Does the Black Women Want Most?
Her greatest challenges are:

A. Getting rid of the dryness,
B. Stopping the excessive breakage, and
C. Getting the hair to grow.

The dryness is mostly responsible for the breakage. The No-Lye Relaxer kits are totally responsible for the dryness. This extreme dryness far exceeds what is normal. The dryness this **Dehydrating Monster** creates is the reason women of color are collectively spending $9 billion every year—it's not because they love the products they are purchasing and using. They are searching for solutions to the dryness, the breakage, and a lack of growth. Nothing is working, and their hair is constantly falling out!

The Testing Phase

All hair care companies test their products to see how well they work before placing the products on the market. This means they are well aware of the dryness the **No-Lye Relaxer** causes and this has been known for many years. The **No-Lye Relaxer** has destroyed so much hair that today the vast majority of black women, regardless of their socioeconomic status, have experienced some degree of hair loss. Many have experienced extreme hair loss. In fact they and their daughters are wearing false hair more today than ever before.

The Real Solution Hair Care System will:

A. Undo the damage with newly grown hair,
B. reverse the dryness,
C. stop the breakage, and
D. get the hair to grow longer than ever.

Its Abilities

As I mentioned earlier, Dudley makes the ONLY PRODUCT capable of reversing this extreme dryness. **Crème Pressing Hairdressing** has the ability to cancel any and all dryness from styling sprays, hot curling, blow drying, roller sets, and, most importantly, the dryness that comes for using the NO-LYE RELAXER. Until now, this type of dryness was impossible to conquer. There is no other product capable of reversing the excessive dryness from the **No-Lye Relaxer** except **Crème Press Hairdressing.**

Intensive Care Extra-Moisturizing Conditioners with Protein!

I know there is no such thing, but the concept is necessary. The types of moisture-producing ingredients in the products matter more than anything else. Most moisturizing conditioners do not work with black hair because they were not designed to tackle the severity of the dryness this **Dehydrating Monster (No-Lye Relaxer)** causes. Also getting moisture into the cortex of the hair is not a matter of depth but rather a matter of retention. In other words, it is the amount of time the moisture remains in the hair that makes the difference. Again the solution is **Crème Press Hairdressing.**

There must be a continuous process that makes the conditioning treatments work. The process of imparting moisture into the hair begins with the application of the **Concentrated Moisturizing Conditioner** that takes place after each shampoo. It must be allowed to remain on the hair for twenty minutes, while you wear a plastic cap and sit under a warm hood dryer. This is a different type of conditioner than what is applied to the hair after it is blown dry. The **Crème Press Hairdressing** is the key in this position of the treatment.

It is commonly thought that the only types of conditioners are lotion-enriched moisture-absorbing humectants. However, the process also requires creamy emollients that will soften and retain moisture in the hair shaft for many days. This is an entirely different type of conditioner than the ones that are applied after each shampoo. This conditioner must be applied after the hair is blown dry. This type of leave-in conditioner hairdressing, moisturizing crème is designed to restore the hair's natural oils and moisture.

The Hair Bends Rather Than Breaks

This hairdressing is concentrated but extremely light. It will not weigh the hair down and will greatly improve the hair's elasticity, **enabling the hair to bend rather than break** during daily styling and combing. The oil content is almost identical, if not lighter than, the natural oils normally secreted from the oil glands.

The 24 Month-Growth Timetable is a weekly Intensive Moisture and Strength Treatment Process. When followed according to directions, this process will:

a) Hydrate and revive dry hair,
b) moisturize and strengthen hair,
c) smooth and seal split ends,
d) detangle and add sheen to hair,
e) repair and rebuild damaged dry hair, and
f) Replenish elasticity, all in an effort to help prevent the hair from breaking.

Many women think that heavy oils are the answer for every hair care problem. Actually, heavy oils are not the answer for any hair care problem. (**Crème Press Hairdressing** has very little oil in its formula.)

This is very important! The idea of the "dime-size portions" is to control the amount of the hairdressing you are applying. Remember, you are not using **Crème Press Hairdressing** for sheen alone. What makes **Crème Press Hairdressing** special is all of the things it does for your hair.

1. The moisture content of **Crème Press Hairdressing** actually repels heavy moisture in the air on a rainy day and even sweat, which are different kinds of moisture that the hair does not need.
2. Then with all of that going on, it conditions the hair with every application. So the key is to use it in very small amounts. If a dime-size portion is too much, use half as much or even a smaller amount.
3. It is the perfect Crème for Pressing and Curling natural hair. This is what it was originally made for.

4. Considering all of the things **Crème Press Hairdressing** can do for your hair, its only job is to "dress the hair." It is a finishing sheen in crème form. You don't need anything else.

In the Salon, when I use Total Control Styling Spray mixed with **Crème Press Hairdressing, it's like** "magic in my hands." With these two products I can make the hair do anything I want the hair to do. They give me **Absolute Control** over the way the hair hold curls, its shape and form, and **Absolute Control** over every aspect of my styling process. With practice you too can perfect the use of every product in this System. Plus the **Crème Press Hairdressing and Styling Spray** conditions the hair with every application.

It is important to remember not to wait until the hair is dry to apply the **Crème Press**. **Crème Press Hairdressing** is to be applied daily to prevent the dry hair from returning.

Cathy Recommends Heavy Oils

The way to know if the hair products you are using are the right ones for your hair is that the right one will AWAYS deliver. The right products will accomplish what you need them to do.

Today it seems as though women want styling the hair to be like "buying fast food." That isn't really possible when it comes to caring for black hair because the hair dictates. Let me explain. The healthier your hair is, the more it will cooperate with styling techniques. Women today are wearing softer looks with much less curl. The hair moves, has bounce, and it is not stuck together with heavy oils and gels that dry hard. Hard hair isn't soft—it looks hard, and that's not the way a woman's hair should look or feel.

The opposite of *DRYNESS* is *MOISTURE*. The very nature of both words has somehow been burned into your psyche. Most women will buy any product with moisture on the label. They will use it every day, but no matter how much they use, their hair is still dry. The products simply do not deliver!

A woman's hair should always be soft to the touch. Moisture in the hair is determined by how soft your hair is, not how oily your hair is. The hair can have no sheen and still be soft. A "greasy look" says "cheap heavy oils," not "sheen," not "moisture," not "softness," not "healthy," and certainly not "beautiful."

I wish I could get black women beyond the obsession for using oil on the hair and beyond the insanity of thinking there is some benefit in getting the hair to shine artificially. It is commonly thought that oil is a cure for "everything" that is wrong with your hair. You wake up every day and apply oil to your hair, on top of the oil from the days and weeks before. Oil is not the determining factor as to whether your hair is healthy or not. Heavy oils will not make it healthy, and the hair doesn't look healthy with tons of oil on it!

How do you know if there is too much oil on your hair?

- If it looks greasy, it's too much!
- If you haven't shampooed after two weeks of applying oil, it's too much!
- If you can squeeze out enough to fry an egg, it's too much!
- If there's enough oil in your hair to share with ten friends, it's too much!
- If you can scratch your scalp and get greasy fingers, it's too much!
- If water rolls right off your hair, it's too much!
- If you've been applying it every day for a month, it's too much!

- If there's a big greasy spot on your pillow, it's too much!
- If it feels like something is crawling on your scalp and that it's filthy, it's too much!
- If there's no lather when you shampoo, it's too much!
- If you smudge your honey's eyeglasses when you hug him, it's too much!
- If you're trying to make false hair look real, and it isn't working, it's too much!
- If what you're using was made for cooking, it's too much!
- If someone can see himself or herself in the shine on your face from the oil flowing everywhere, it's too much!
- If the oil is screaming back at you when you look in the mirror, it's too much!
- If the oil is running down your neck, it's too much!
- If you scratch your scalp and your nails are black, that's just filthy!

I have been in this business over thirty years, and to this day I have never used oil of any kind on anyone's hair. If heavy oils are so important to hair, why is it that black women are the only women who use it? Putting heavy oils on your hair serves no purpose. I'm speaking of the bottles of heavy oils and jars of grease you buy off the shelves.

Manufacturers of superior hair care products realize the distinctive difference in the types of oil-producing ingredients, and they select the right oils from plants, nuts, and other materials that are beneficial to the overall health of your hair. The idea of shiny hair is a natural way of thinking, and yes, the hair is healthier when it has shine. The shine, however, is from a healthy cuticle layer and no oils are involved.

When it comes to selecting hair care products, trust the Professionals: stylists and chemists who make **High Quality** hair care products. NEVER trust the advice of a nonprofessional, especially one without a license and a minimum of ten years of experience. Cathy may recommend heavy oils, but Cathy doesn't know what she's talking about.

You've Searched Everywhere for Answers to these Questions:

- How do I get my hair to grow?
- How can I chemically relax my hair and keep it on my head?
- How do I stop the shedding and breakage?
- How do I select the best hair care products for my hair?
- What's the best chemical relaxer?
- What are conditioners all about, and how do they work?
- Is it possible to use a Lye Relaxer with no burns?
- How do I use styling sprays and hairdressing for stronger curls?
- How do I get sheen without a heavy oily look?
- What about shampoos, do they matter?
- Why is my hair so dry, and how do I end the dryness once and for all?
- No-Lye Relaxers, are they any good?
- Are the new relaxers made with Calcium Hydroxide, Lithium, and Sodium Hydroxide right for my hair?

There are probably many more questions you need answered, and **Shamboosie's Hair Wellness Approach to Hair Growth** was created to put an end to your search. We have made sure you understand all you need to know about your hair. In this book you will **Discover the REAL Secrets of Growing Longer, Healthier Hair and** that's my promise. The incredible collection of hair care products I recommend were designed to address all of your hair care needs.

Black people naturally have very dry hair and skin. But the dryness that comes from using the No-Lye Relaxer is **extraordinary**. Therefore, the product needed to control this dryness must also be extraordinary. **As I've mentioned,** I have discovered what I believe is the best product to combat this dryness: **Crème Press Hairdressing from Dudley Products.** It is a very light crème made with just a hint of refined oils and other unique moisturizing properties that are perfect for your hair. (It's important to remember not to wait until the hair is dry to apply this product. **Crème Press Hairdressing** is to be applied daily to prevent the dry hair from ever returning.)

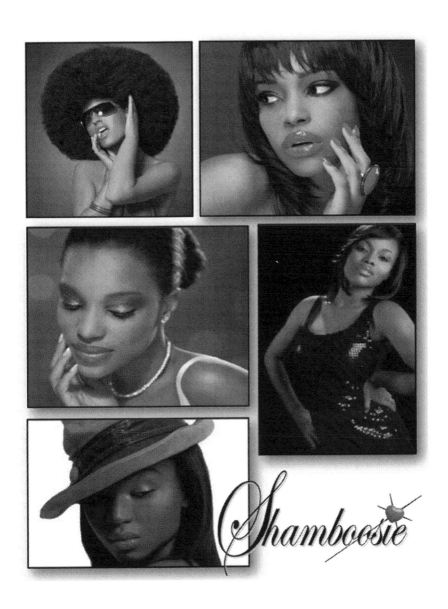

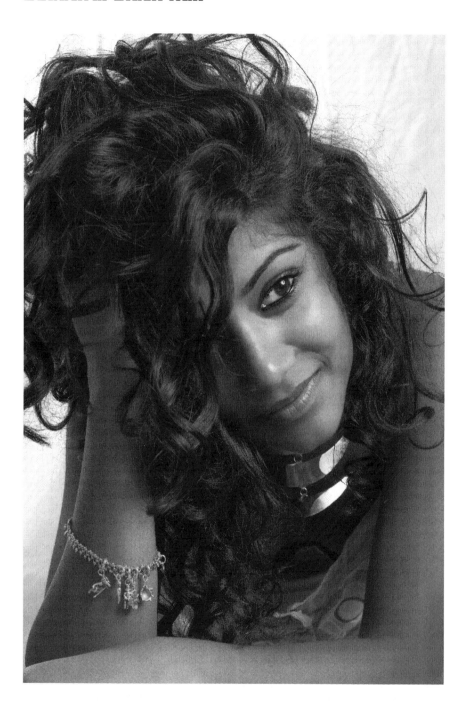

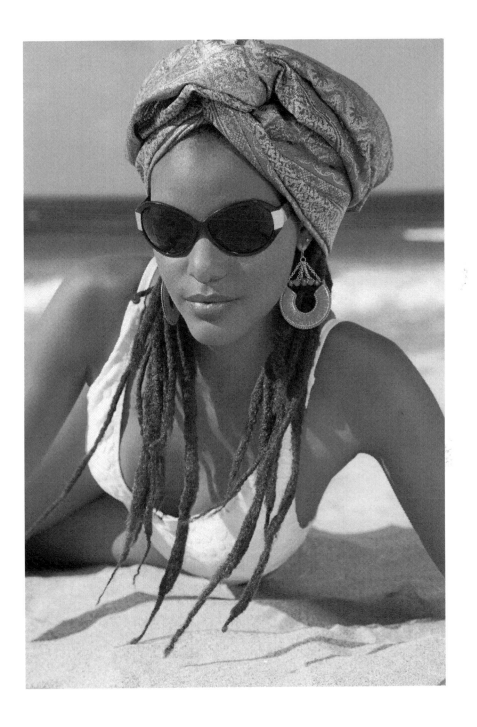

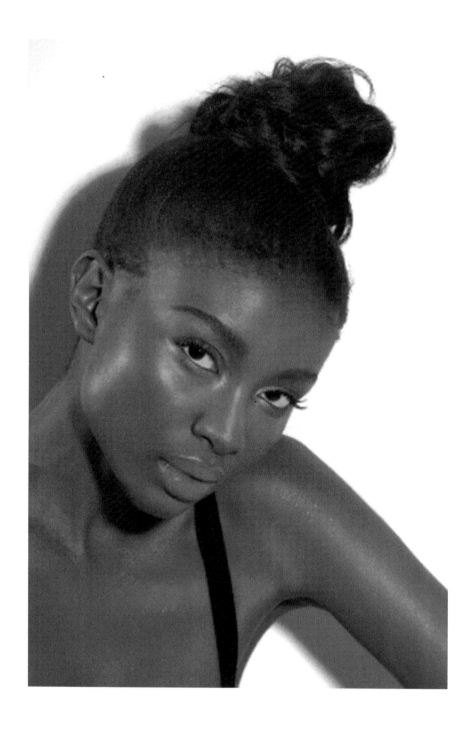

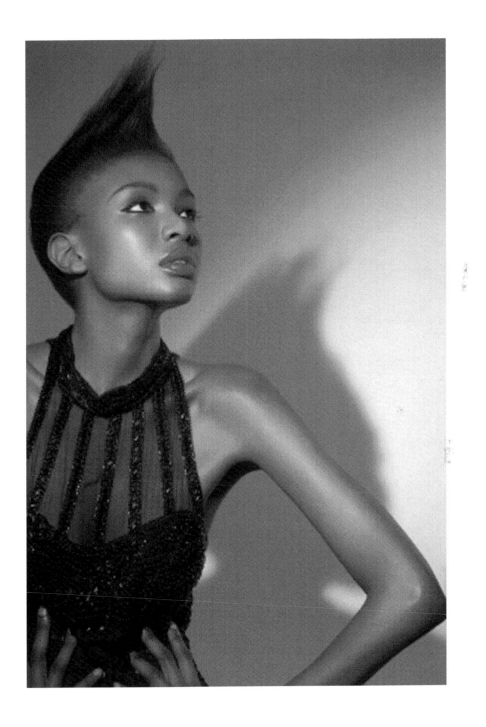

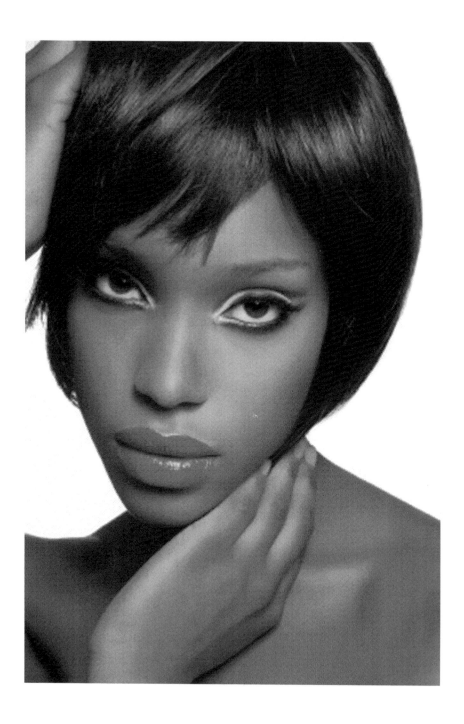

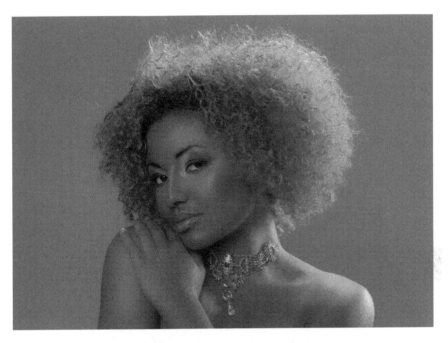

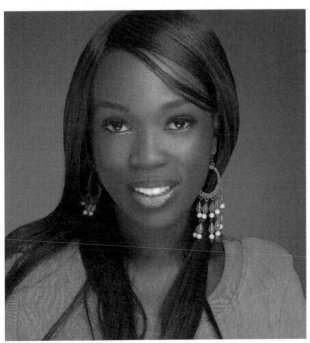

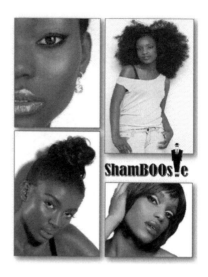

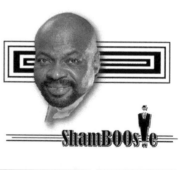

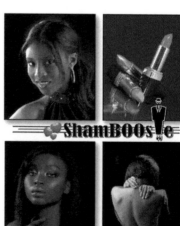

Chapter 5

The Amazing New Ceramic Flat Iron

MASTER the Art of Using this Professional Tool of the Trade

Ceramic Flat Irons are the newest, most advanced professional styling tools, and they are simply amazing. Keep in mind when you purchase this tool it must have a *ceramic* plate. This is a much better approach to pressing natural hair and hair that has been treated with Chemical Relaxer and/or Permanent Hair color. Add just a film or light coating of **Crème Press Conditioning Hairdressing** to every strand, spray on some **Styling Spray,** and let the magic begin. The Flat Iron has two ceramic plates that maintain even temperature. They create a gentler, softer heat that protects the hair's luster and moisture and prevents scorching of the hair.

A ShamBOOsie Tip: I place a quarter-size portion of **Crème Press Conditioning Hairdressing** on the back of my left hand (I am right-handed) and curl hair with the flat iron/curlers in my right hand. I will use my thumb and the first two fingers of my right hand to apply a very thin, very light film of **Crème Press Conditioning Hairdressing** to both the top side and the bottom side of each section of the hair. I comb the hair with a fine-tooth rattail comb from scalp to the ends of each section of hair. Then I spray on some medium-hold styling spray and place the Ceramic Flat Iron on the section of hair parallel to the parting. I turn the Flat Iron slightly toward me, and in one continuous movement, gently pull it through the section of hair. **The finish is smooth, silky, and so soft to the touch.**

When you apply **Crème Press Conditioning Hairdressing,** you greatly increase the protection level of your hair from all forms of heat damage, plus you add longer-lasting softness and a brilliant subtle sheen. You can straighten or press hair of any length with the one-inch plates. The flat, heated plates actually press the hair, and the ceramic surface allows the iron to slide through the hair with ease. They also feature beveled or rounded edges for turning the ends of the hair up or under. These are the styling trends of today's creative, lightly textured, youthful looks. Women of color are wearing softer, smoother, straighter looks that are much easier to manage. That is the reason it's so important to GROW your hair as long as possible, and this book will help you do that. One of the most attractive advantages of the flat iron is that it is easy for most anyone to use. This newest technology permits faster styling that reduces the hair's exposure to heat and dryness.

Acquiring Real Solutions is all about Real GROWTH and to accomplish this, one must master the Art of using superior Hair Care products, as well as superior Professional Tools such as the new **ceramic flat iron,** which offers maximum control over the styling process. The heat distribution of the ceramic plates is unmatched, steady, and there when you need it. There are separate heating systems for each plate, 170 watts of power for fast heat up and instant heat recovery after working with each section of hair. The unit heats up in less than sixty seconds from the time the switch is turned on. The best and most professional flat irons will cost between, $90-$160. You can find them as low as $40, but these will not last as long or work as well. The size of plate to look for is five-eighths to one inch wide. This size allows you to work with hair of most lengths from three inches to everything longer. Flat irons are very portable, and they are great to touch up your curls after a work-out. Steer clear of flat irons with variable heat settings knobs. You only want to turn it on and off! When the iron heats to a certain point, it will maintain an even temperature. Once you use a flat iron you may never go back to curlers!

Using Your CHI Ceramic Hair Straightening Flat Iron

There are still many of the OLD flat irons on the market, these are not the newest technology. I suggest you buy a one-inch **CHI ceramic flat iron**; it's the one ShamBOOsie uses but there are less expensive flat irons. Whatever you do, don't go into the store and ask for a flat iron. You need a **ceramic flat iron.** It will sell for about $90.00 online; Keyword: **CHI ceramic flat irons**. Remember this is a FLAT surface not a curling iron, and it is not a metal flat surface. Just flip the iron slightly toward yourself, and hold the position throughout each section of hair.

Step 1: First make sure the hair is completely dry. This will protect the hair from the heat! If the hair is not very kinky, you can also use the new **ceramic flat irons** to hot press this texture of hair. You want to get the hair as straight as possible during the drying process. This will require spraying setting lotion on all the hair, combing it through. Use a towel to remove most of the moisture from the hair, and allow the hair to rest for about five minutes before drying.

Step 2: Separate the hair into five or six sections and blow each section dry. If any of the sections become dry before you get the chance to blow it dry, spray a light mist of setting lotion to dampen the hair. **The hair MUST be dried from damp to dry and straight.**

Step 3: Coat every strand of your hair before starting with a heat-protective, cream hairdressing. **ShamBOOsie's Miracle Hair**

Softening Methodology is to take a dime-size portion of Crème Press Hairdressing and rub it between the psalms of your hands. Rub the hands together rapidly to create friction and heat. This will cause the hairdressing to become very thin. Cover your hands and between your fingers with the hairdressing, so that application is easier. It only takes a very thin, very light coat of the product on each strand to work. You can always apply more where and when needed, even throughout the day. Use a very light, gentle touch during the application. Never squeeze the hair between the ceramic plates. Apply the Crème Press every day so that the hair NEVER becomes dry. Spray on some medium hold styling spray to help the hair hold all day long.

Step 4: Start wherever you are most comfortable, since you have to manage the hair daily. If your hair is four to ten inches long, you will probably wear it soft with very little curl. Take a two-inch section of hair and gently place the iron on the hair as close to the scalp as possible. DON'T USE ANY PRESSURE; use a gentle touch. You want the iron to glide easily. Then quickly and gently in one motion turn the iron toward you just slightly and hold it in this position as you pull iron down the full length of hair. It works like putting a bend or a circle in a ribbon to make a bow. NEVER buy a **ceramic flat iron** with adjustable heat setting knobs. The **CHI ceramic flat iron** comes preset.

Step 5: Comb to style as usual. To get the best results from your ceramic flat iron, clean the iron daily with a wet cloth. Never allow the iron to become dirty. It is easier to clean while it is still hot, so use caution when wiping the flat iron clean. Achieving perfect results is what it's all about, and ShamBOOsie's Methodology will help you do it right and safely.

In order to achieve the best result every time from your flat iron you MUST always shampoo, condition your hair very well, at least three or four times, every two or three days for ten days, with the EXACT and perfect conditioning products. It will make all the difference.

ShamBOOsie's Hot Tip: Never HOLD the flat iron on the hair, in one place for too long. The iron MUST always be in motion while on the hair. You should only need to pass the flat iron through the hair once when you get the hang of it, and never more than twice. This is especially true for color-treated hair. Make sure the hair is very strong and conditioned well if you intend to Hot Press or Hot Curl hair with permanent color in it. Remember to keep the iron in motion when it in the hair. It takes only forty-five seconds to heat up.

You Will Learn: Creating Perfect Styles as You Go

Even long wigs and weaves can easily be managed with the new ceramic flat irons. I will be producing a DVD soon after this book is released that will show you how to do it.

Everyone is doing flips. There is a different look with every length and style of hair. It is a simple and easy way to bend the hair that is versatile and looks good on anyone. You can also use the ceramic flat iron to press your little one's hair. This is the perfect way to avoid using a chemical relaxer on her hair. If you're going to press her hair, use a little more of the **Crème Press Hairdressing** because it will aid in the straightening process and add even more softness to the hair. To achieve perfect hairstyle results, start now taking your time and go slowly. You will have the hang of this new styling concept in just a few weeks.

A ShamBOOsie Tip:

Every strand of hair must receive an application of the **Crème Press.** I cannot stress the importance of applying **Crème Press** during the pressing process and daily afterwards. Sectioning the hair will make this process easier and ensure all areas are covered. Start in the back left or right side of the head and at the bottom of the section.

Styling Concepts

Today, smoother, softer looks, with little or no curls, are popular. If you want to wear the hair off the face, before the hair is completely dry, push the hair toward the back of the head while fanning it with hot air from the blow dryer. Fanning the heat will help to move the air through the hair, causing separation, which allows the hair to dry softer and faster. To add volume on top, blow the hair forward down toward the face until it's dry. Then comb the hair back toward the back of the head and with one hand, push the hair forward.

If you want the hair on the right side to move back away from the face, over the ear, and to lie close to the scalp, push it in that direction and dry the hair so that it will fall that way. Simply visualize what you want the hair to do, one section, and even one curl or bend, at a time. Hairstyling is just that simple and easier today than ever before. The hair is dried "on base" when it exits the scalp and immediately lies down on the scalp in any direction.

A Hair Pressing Issue

The hot pressing method of straightening the hair is one of the oldest methods of straightening overly curly hair. It's amazing that *the art of pressing the hair* is resurging in popularity. It is being used as an alternative to chemical relaxers. Many of you think that chemical relaxers are making your hair fall out. You are right, but the problem is the **No-Lye Relaxer** and the person applying it to your hair. There is an excellent chemical relaxer that is safer to use, and it actually improves the texture of your hair during the process. Many women who don't want their hair relaxed but don't want to wear it natural either is opting to have the hair hot pressed and curled.

Younger stylists know very little about the art of pressing the hair. So it would be wise to find a stylist that has been in the business for a while. See a stylist with the ability to skillfully use a hot comb, or you could lose a lot of hair. Hot combs are made in two sizes and two shapes. I prefer the small comb for doing most of the work; these are the ones with slightly curved thin teeth. They allow you to get as close to the scalp as possible without burning. The small comb is for work in tight areas and for working with hair that is very short. The larger comb is for longer, thicker hair, but a professional can use either one and do the job well.

Techniques for Pressing the Hair

- This is another process that requires two people, which means you should not press your own hair unless you already know how to do so properly. The possibility of scalp burns increases when you do it yourself.
- The hair can be pressed in small sections, or, if you are good at it, you may start anywhere on the head, as long as all of the hair has been pressed when all is said and done.
- Remove any distractions. Pressing hair is an "eyes-on" technique that requires concentration. You do not want to talk to anyone or watch TV while pressing hair.
- The comb is very hot, so please be very careful, and take your time.
- The pressing comb should be hot, but not hot enough to burn the hair.
- Hold the ends of hair with your free hand, and place the teeth of the hot comb into the hair about a one-quarter inch off the scalp.
- Keep the comb in place, and rotate the back of the comb down, as close to the scalp as possible, without touching the scalp. The pressing or straightening of the hair is done with the back of the

hot comb. The teeth of the hot comb simply separate the strands of the hair.

- Pull the comb through the hair once or twice to *"soft press"* the hair, and two to four times to *"hard press"* the hair. The Crème Press will leave the hair smooth and silky but not oily.
- After all the hair has been hot pressed, you can either roller set the hair or hot curl to style. If you decide to hot curl the hair, spray the hair lightly with the styling spray and curl as usual.
- The hair should be pressed every week to maintain.

Pressing Color, Curled, and Chemically Relaxed Hair

The BREAKING point! If there is permanent hair color, a curl, or a chemical relaxer in your hair, DO NOT hot press the hair using a straightening comb. This applies even if you intend to press only the new growth. You will burn out and lose ALL the hair! This will cause the hair to break and fall out. The heat from the hot iron will burn through the chemically treated hair and cause breakage at the *line of demarcation* where the new growth and the previously relaxed hair meet.

Properly heating the pressing comb or Marcel curling irons is the key to getting the desired finished look. This could be very difficult to do at home. Heating the Marcel irons on top of your kitchen stove is very different than using a stove made for this purpose. On the kitchen stove, the irons will always get too hot, and the heat will be uneven and more intense. This will burn the hair right off the head.

How to Take Complete Control of the Heat

- Fold a cloth hand towel three times and wet it with cold water. Be sure to leave some of the liquid in the towel. It should be very wet but not dripping. Place the towel near the stove for easy access.

- The first time the iron is placed in the stove, it will take about two minutes to heat to a temperature hot enough to curl hair.
- The way to test the heat is to lay the barrel of the curling iron on the towel soaked with cold water before putting the iron into the hair. This way you can make sure the iron is not too hot but is sufficiently hot for curling.
- The key to controlling the heat is in *the sound of the iron touching the towel* soaked with cold water.
- If you listen carefully, the sound you will hear when a curling iron is too hot for curling, is *a blistering sound* like dropping cold water into a hot pan.
- If you hear "*a slight hissing sound*," it means the iron is safe to begin curling the hair. The iron will only be hot enough for creating about three curls before you'll need to reheat it. It should only take twenty to thirty seconds to reheat but be sure to test the iron *every* time. The twenty-thirty seconds should be just enough time to section the hair, comb the section, and add a smidgen of Crème Press and Styling Spray. Comb through the section, and then curl that section of hair.
- *Important:* Marcel irons are for *professional use.* I do not suggest using them at home, unless you know how to use them properly.

Cooling the Curling Irons

If you continue rubbing the iron on the wet towel, it will quiet the sound, cooling the iron in the process. If the sound goes away completely, the iron is too cool to curl the hair, and must be reheated and cooled again. Getting the iron to the right temperature for curling will require some practice. Remember, you want to hear "*a slight hissing sound,*" which will mean the iron is safe to use. Occasionally, you may need to replenish the cold water in the towel.

- *Never leave the irons on a hot stove unattended.* The irons will become too hot to handle. If you were to touch them, you won't be touching anything else for about three months. If the irons are accidentally left on the stove too long, do not touch them with your bare hands. Use a thick, folded, *wet* towel to remove the irons.

- Never put overheated irons in cold water to cool. This will cause *warping*, and the irons will be useless.
- Put the irons in a safe place to cool, not near food. Be sure they are out of the reach of children and away from anything that could catch fire.

Do Not Touch to Test

Never touch the stove or the irons to determine if they are hot enough for pressing or curling hair. Do not touch the stove even if you know it is unplugged or cold. If the iron is hot you will never be able to touch it quick enough not to burn yourself. There are two ways to turn off the stove and the curling irons—turn the switch to the *off* position, and unplug both the stove and the curling irons.

A ShamBOOsie Tip: After your hair has been given a cut of your choice, here are a few tips that will help you when styling your hair at home. Remember to set aside enough time and then take your time and practice.

Drying the Hair

When blow-drying always dry different sections of hair in the direction you intend to style. If you want soft pieces of hair on the face and forehead, use the following procedure. Using a fine-tooth comb, dry those small sections with the base as close to the scalp and skin as possible. Simply lay the hair down on the face and dry the hair.

If all the hair is to be styled forward from the crown and down the back of the head, blow-dry the hair down and from the crown to both sides, and blow the top forward. Curl the hair in the same direction in "pie-shaped" sections or pick up the hair and curl it. Whatever type of curl you choose, the hairstyle should turn out well. The curling should begin around the hairline and face of each front section, and work your way to a point in the crown. The hair on the face should be curled softly or slightly bent, so it will lie on the face.

I recommend using **Dudley's Crème Press Hairdressing** and **Dudley's Total Control** (spray). I have found them to work the best for the hot iron set. Curling with these products will ensure that the curls hold and last three to four days without having to roll, set, or re-curl the hair. Whenever re-curling is necessary, simply repeat the process, and use a small portion of **Crème Press** daily.

Blow-Drying the Hair

The reason hair is often "puffed up" after drying is because often you are in a hurry to get the hair dry. Also there is a chance that most of the hair air dries on its own. It is important to take the time to do it the right way.

ShamBOOsie Suggests: Allow enough time to dry your hair properly, and slow the process down. You do not have to dry your hair in the first ten minutes, so take your time. Keep your eye on what you are doing. Start by spraying in premixed setting lotion, and then dry the hair in small sections.

You may need to spray a little more setting lotion occasionally to keep the hair damp but not wet. The hair will dry straighter and smoother because you are drying from damp to dry. Any unwanted wave or curl in the hair will be very difficult to get out after you have allowed the hair to dry on its own.

95

Beautiful Black Hair

ShamBOOsie Suggests:

- Clip or pin up the hair that is not being dried to keep it out away from the flow of the heat.
- If a section of hair air-dries before you are able blow it dry, spray in a little water or setting lotion on the hair as you go.
- It is best to use a small plastic spray bottle about two inches tall that sprays a light mist. It will allow you to dampen the hair rather than wet the hair.
- Remember, drying the hair from wet to dry is the key to getting it straight. Use the dryer's comb attachment, put a little tension on the hair as you dry it, and direct the heat only toward the hair that is being dried

Getting the Hair at the Nape to Lie Down

When the hair is very short in the back, getting it to lie down is easier at times than others. Keep the very short hair freshly relaxed (about every three to four weeks) but only in those very short areas. The hair will grow, and in as little as two weeks there will be *new growth*. The *new growth* will be different in texture. It will have some curl, which tends to push the short hair out. The new hair simply will not stay down.

When the hair has been relaxed, add setting gel. Smooth the hair in the back with a fine-tooth comb, while removing all excess setting gel. Tie the hair down with paper neck strips and allow the hair to dry completely. After the hair is dry, add a smidgen of Crème Press to all the hair, and style as usual.

Making the Curls Hold and Last

When the hair is relaxed, it loses its ability to naturally hold a curl. Hairstylists take note. *No matter what style you give a client, if the style doesn't hold, the client has wasted her money, and you have done a lot of work for nothing.*

96

ShamBOOsie Suggests: Select a good spray but not one that creates *a firm hold.* Choose a styling cream or hairdressing that is not oily. Oil causes the hair to shine for about one hour before the set falls out. This is because oil expands with the heat from the scalp and will soften the set, causing all the curls to fall.

By the way, *never use grease on your hair.* I recommend **Crème Press Hairdressing**, and **Total Control** holding spray both from Dudley Products. They are the best.

- First, the styling **Crème Press** is applied lightly to all of the hair, in dime-size portions with the palm of the hands. Use a very light touch, apply sparingly, and be sure every strand is covered. Use as much of the crème as you need but only in dime-size portions, so as to not use too much.
- Next, spray all of the hair generously with the Total Control spray, and comb through the hair with a large-tooth comb. Dry the hair completely, and apply extra Crème Press where needed while curling. In most cases, the curls will be soft to the touch but will hold for two to three days or longer. I have had many clients whose curls would last a week and longer without rolling or re-curling the hair.
- Remember to position each curl, and allow the finished curled set to cool completely before combing out. Do not comb after each curl. Always use a very wide-tooth comb that has three to four large teeth for the comb out, and comb the hair in as few strokes as possible. This will allow several strands of the hair to hold together, supporting one another, and the curls will last longer. Using a fine-tooth comb will cause too much separation of the hair strands, and the curls in the set will fall out.

Beautiful Black Hair

Important: Be gentle with your grip on the hair. This will allow the heated curling iron to do all the work. If sticking occurs, loosen the hair from the iron with the tail of the rat-tail comb, and continue curling. The curling irons are designed so that the roundness of the irons and the heat will get the job done. No pressure is ever needed, so be gentle. The rest is art.

The Right Way to Hot Press the Hair

Much has been written about black people wearing their hair natural and chemical free. Some say that it is an expression of African pride and heritage. I have always wondered why a professional hairstylist would suggest that one should wear his or her hair *natural* because as long as it's worn natural, the less the client needs to have it serviced. Pressing and curling or wearing the hair natural may be chemical-free options for some people. However, relaxers, curls, and other chemicals will continue to have a wide appeal. Let's face it, the natural look does not appeal to every woman.

In "the old days," when pressing her daughters' hair, sometimes Mom would put too much oil on the hair. Then the hot iron would melt the grease, causing it to also become hot. The grease would "*pop*" onto the scalp and cause real pain.

What made the whole ordeal even more threatening was that whenever Mom would get a little too close with that iron, although she was being very careful, she would accidentally burn the scalp, forehead, the ears or and neck. Each time she would say how sorry she was and then tell you to "*sit still and stop squirming so much.*" You could hardly wait until the whole thing was over. Pressing and curling the hair should never be such a painful experience.

Using Styling Spray

Styling spray will help to hold the set or the curls when used the right way. However, when used alone, it can leave the hair very hard and dry to the touch, which is not good for women of color; you already have enough dryness to deal with. Styling sprays contain some alcohol, and this alone dries the hair out. The makers of styling sprays for use on black hair realize the alcohol content must be at a minimum. This is probably the only good thing I can say about a product that was *made for use on black hair.*

Crème Press is mentioned many times earlier in this and other chapters because it is so essential to the survival of your hair. When hot curling with Marcel irons, **Crème Press** and **Total Control** are a winning combination.

Hard Pressing and Soft Pressing

A *Hard pressing* will last about a week and a *soft pressing* will last two to three days.

Pressing the Hair: This is How We Do It

1. Shampoo and condition the hair twice or three times as needed.
2. Towel dry the hair to remove as much water as possible.
3. Spray in some setting lotion to soften the hair. The setting lotion will soften the hair and close the cuticle layer, making the hair easier to comb.
4. Detangle the hair using a wide-tooth comb. Separate hair into as many small sections as possible.
5. Pin each small section up and out of the way. This will make blow-drying the hair much easier. Begin combing the first section toward the scalp, starting with the ends of the hair. Use a very wide-tooth comb to remove all of the tangles.
6. Next, using a blow dryer with a comb attachment, dry each section as straight as possible.

Important: Water in the hair will *air dry* quickly because there is nowhere else for the water to go. The hair cannot absorb the excess water. The problem with this is that whatever natural curl or wave pattern is in the hair will surface when the hair dries. This curl will be impossible to remove when you blow the hair dry, without wetness or water moisture in the hair. It shouldn't be dripping wet, but it should be wet not dry. You want to make sure the section of hair you are working with has some moisture in it before you begin drying it.

You also want to keep moisture in the hair to be able to dry it from wet to dry. This is the only way to remove the curl and get the hair straight. You will need a comb attachment on the end of the dryer or use a regular comb to hold the hair straight until it is dry.

Drying the hair from wet to dry will help to remove as much of the wave or curl from the hair as possible. This will not be possible if the hair is allowed to *air dry*. So you will need a small spray bottle that sprays a light mist of moisture or water, to slightly wet the hair if it dries before you have the chance to blow it dry. Begin drying around the face, and completely dry each small section before moving on to the next. The key to doing it well is in taking your time. Set aside enough time to do it the right way.

Slow the process down. When your arms get tired (and they will), take a break, watch a little TV, or have something to drink. Then spray a little water and start again. You can do this as many times as needed.

When all of the hair is dry, use **Crème Press** in dime-size portions. Apply to all of the hair, from scalp to end, and be sure the crème is on all of the hair. Then section the hair into as many small sections as possible to press and straighten the hair.

Let's Press Hair

- Starting around the face, pick up each one-quarter inch section of hair.
- Apply a little more **Crème Press** to every section before pressing.
- Take your time and be very careful. This is a very hot iron, and to do a good job, this hot comb will have to be placed very close to the scalp.
- Place the hot comb in the hair as close to the scalp as possible. With a little pressure, press and pull the hot comb through to the ends of the hair. You may need to do this a couple of times to get the hair silky smooth and straight from the scalp to the ends.
- Move to the next section and repeat the same process until all the hair has been pressed and straightened. When using any hot iron or hot comb, it is very important to do all of the work with the tip of the irons. This will give you more control of the iron and of the hair. Now get with it, *"press the issue!"*

Grooming Natural Hair

Before any grooming enters the picture there is a complication. Depending on the hair's natural style, shampooing and conditioning the hair can be very difficult. The problem is that when you are wearing braids, cornrows, and other natural styles, including synthetic hair, there is the possibility of locs becoming undone or braids slipping loose and coming out. Perhaps you think that if your braids are not real hair, it doesn't make sense to shampoo or condition them? This is absolutely wrong. Since your real hair is also a part of the equation, it becomes the very reason a good shampoo and a very good conditioner is vital to maintain its health. The process is a constant, which means you must shampoo and condition regularly—there are no exceptions. In terms of the natural hair, locs or otherwise, being long, thick and more difficult to clean doesn't change a thing.

101

Beautiful Black Hair

Perhaps you are thinking that rinsing shampoos and cream conditioner will be troublesome to manage or that creamy conditioners will cause a buildup on the hair and scalp. You are both right and wrong, but it doesn't change a thing. You still have to shampoo and condition regularly with very good products, no exceptions.

The reason some shampoos and conditioners leave a buildup is because they coat the hair. They are designed to make you think they have done wonders for your hair, and they have corrected many of the problems with weak, lifeless, and dry hair. These are mostly cheap products so stay away from them. The solution is quality hair care products. They can be removed as easily as they are applied, plus they will keep the hair as healthy, strong, and as beautiful as possible. To not shampoo and condition regularly will result in problems with your hair such as dryness, hair breakage, and damage to the cuticle and cortex layer. The thing to remember is that once the hair is damaged it cannot be undone.

Less Curl Is Better

Somewhere between natural hair and chemically relaxed hair is a concept called *Texturizing the Hair*. I wanted to add this chemical technique to this chapter because many women already find themselves with curl or wave in the hair they can't remove, as with what is left from using the No-Lye Relaxer. The ceramic iron and Crème Press is the solution. But if you are using only a Lye Relaxer removing some of the curl while *leaving some of curl* gives the hair more body. (I'm only talking about leaving 15-25 percent of the natural curl.) This approach to chemically relaxing the hair leaves the hair with more bounce, more life, more strength, and more GROWTH.

This is a true story: My client, Brittanie Monique, returned to the salon the week after getting her retouch, complaining that the relaxer I gave her the week before didn't completely straighten her hair. (I have seen this many times over many years). *This is not a matter to complain about!* This is a very good thing to do for your hair. It is really the way the hair should always be relaxed. This is called *Texturizing the Hair.* If your goal is hair that is soft, strong, full of body, and full of life, then it makes perfect sense to leave a percentage of the natural curl in the hair.

The life of the hair is in the natural bonds, that part of the hair that is destroyed during the chemical process. To leave some of the curl in the hair leaves some of it life in the hair. It's actually one of the best things you can do for your hair. Use of a comb attachment with your blow dryer and a ceramic flat iron will take care of the rest of the curl. This is where the magic of your Crème Press Hairdressing and your styling spray comes into play.

A ShamBOOsie Chemical Tip

The idea of leaving curl for body and life in the hair is only true and will only happen if the only kind of chemical in your hair is a *Conditioning Lye Relaxer.* The higher the quality *Conditioning Lye Relaxer,* the better condition your hair will be in afterward. It is not such a good thing if the chemical in your hair is *No-Lye Relaxer,* for obvious reasons.

A *Conditioning Lye Relaxer* application will leave the natural bonds of your hair with the ability to continue having an effect on the overall health of your hair, by remaining soft to the touch. The conditioners will have a greater chance of keeping the hair healthy. Your hair must always be able to absorb moisture from the conditioners and hairdressing. This will not be possible with a No-Lye Relaxer. Each additional application of the *Conditioning Lye Relaxer,* which MUST take place every six, seven, or eight weeks, will remove a little more of the natural curl. Eventually the hair will become completely relaxed.

This is not the case with the *No-Lye Relaxer*. One application of the *No-Lye Relaxer* will completely neutralize the natural bonds of the hair, rendering each recurring retouch ineffective. If you don't remove all the curl the first time around, you won't get a second chance. It will leave the hair unhealthy and remove all of the hair's moisture. This will cause the hair to become *unnaturally and severely DRY*. It will also weaken the hair and rob it of its body and life. This is never a good thing!

Your hair should have a lovely wavy texture at this point. . It will be very easy to remove the remainder of the curl later with a ceramic flat iron. The latest ceramic flat irons available today are the preferred hot tools for black hair. Don't forget to always use **Crème Press Hairdressing** to protect the hair from the heat.

When I joined the staff of JC Penney Salons, suddenly this veteran of the hair care business was working with white (Caucasian) hair mostly, which was like moving to a new town. However, I was very excited about the possibilities because I had spent most of my career working with black hair. The difference was that I didn't have to deal with Chemically Relaxing Hair because most of the Caucasian women had straight hair. The other difference was the use of new types of hair styling products. There were some products that I use on black hair that I was able to use on white hair as well, such as *styling sprays*. But I could not use any type of oil, as white hair cannot handle oil of any type.

So I began looking for *finishing products* made specifically for white hair. High quality *conditioners* and *shampoos* are about the same for everyone's hair. So they were easiest for me to come up with. I wanted something to help lock in the curls and something that would give the hair a natural shine without *OIL*. I visited another salon in the mall to consult with the stylists there. They were eager to share their knowledge and willing to answer my questions. When I left that salon I went shopping for hair care and hair finishing products.

Being the new kid on the block at JC Penney, I had plenty of time to watch instructional DVDs, and practice the things I saw on those DVDs. I spent two weeks, learning to perfect the use of the new products I had on hand, using the six mannequins in the salon. JC Penney required their salon staff to attend classes on haircutting and other related client services, and I was a sponge eager to soak up all that I could learn. I could barely wait to get a few "living dolls" in my chair to try out some of the new tricks I had been practicing.

The point I am stressing here is the vital importance of using the highest quality tools and Hair Care Products. I spent years studying under some of the top stylists and instructors in the business, and I have spent hundreds of hours honing my skills. Every product and tool that I use is the best that money can buy. I own over 1,000 combs and brushes and over 1,000 rollers and perm rods—all of the highest quality.

When it comes to selecting Hair CARE Products, each product in my possession MUST perform; it MUST accomplish all that I need it to do. If I need to STOP the hair from breaking, the perfect Conditioners MUST work every time without fail. My clients depend on me getting everything right, and I cannot let them down. So if you use the products I use, the way I tell you to use them, you will get the EXACT results.

Beautiful Black Hair

When I purchased a **CHI ceramic flat iron,** it felt like the day I went to pick up a pair of cutting sheers some twenty years earlier. That day when I got the call that my Hair Cutting Shears had arrived, I got dressed up in a suit and tie. My new Cutting Shears were *Joewell Haircutting Shears*—a good balance between value and performance. The choice of shears is very personal for each stylist, but I reach for these when I need to get the best cut possible.

Apart from the obvious performance potential, there are two core principles that separate **Joewell Haircutting Shears** from others on the market. One principle is that certain ideals should never be compromised. The second is that the Highest Standards possible are worth any sacrifice to maintain. These principals are based on a desire for a certain kind of purity and having faith in an unshakable ethic not tied to trends or to anyone's opinion. **Joewell Haircutting Shears** were made for professionals that understand these principles and who share my passion for a supremely competent tool. For hair-stylists who demand this kind of experience, there is no substitute. My first pair cost $350.00, and the price goes up from there.

I remember the day that I thought to myself, "I must have a *CHI Ceramic Flat Iron,* and I must perfect the use of this amazing tool." It is never about cost with **ShamBOOsie**; it is always about quality and getting only the best results. With this tool, you don't have to get your hair "bone straight" using a Chemical Relaxer. You can have your hair relaxed just partially. In fact, the hair will be much healthier this way, unless you want your hair really straight. It's your choice. It is my wish that you wear your hair any way you decide—it's Ladies' Choice!

Chapter 6

ShamBOOsie's Bronze Beauty Emporium

You will never GROW and maintain the health of your hair using inferior, inadequate, deficient, low-priced, inexpensive, bargain-basement, substandard, shoddy black hair products! Below is ShamBOOsie's personal, in Salon List of Hair Care Products. These are the only products he will have on hand and in his product supply room for Services and Retailing. ShamBOOsie will ONLY use **Crème Press Hairdressing & Pressing Crème.** The list and purpose of the Hair Care Products are those things that are what's best for every purpose in caring for your hair. This is Most Important! In this book I want to give you two choices of Quality Hair Care Products from two Manufacturers—**Nexxus Products and Dudley's Products.**

This Is Your Formula for Success:

ShamBOOsie's Hair Wellness Approach to Hair Growth equals the EXACT and Accurate Methods of Application for the Chemical LYE Relaxer. Practice makes perfect; if the EXACT Hair Care System, a Moisturizing Conditioner, a Moisturizing Conditioning Shampoo, and most importantly, a Moisturizing Conditioning Hairdressing is used often and correctly, you'll get the PROMISED RESULTS.

Beautiful Black Hair

If You Come Into ShamBOOsie's Beauty Parlor

I would first examine your hair to determine what condition your hair is in and what it needs to be in its best possible condition. Then I would shampoo your hair with **Therappe Shampoo** and give you a Conditioner Treatment with **Humectress Moisturizing Conditioner!** The Conditioner would remain on your hair for a full twenty-five to thirty minutes before I would rinse it out. I would expect you back in the Salon in five days for a second Conditioner Treatment with **Humectress Moisturizing Conditioner!** After the Conditioner Treatment I would spray on some **Fantastic Body Setting Lotion** and GENTLY detangle your hair one section at a time.

Next I would use a round brush to Blow Dry your hair, directing the hair to fall in the EXACT position I need the hair to fall—on the face, off the face, or straight up off the scalp to give the hair more body and movement. Every strand would be covered with **Crème Press Hairdressing** to protect it from the heat of my ceramic flat iron or my curling irons. Then I would lightly spray on some **Styling Spray because** when the **Crème Press Hairdressing** and the **Styling Spray** come together with my **ceramic flat iron,** it is MAGIC.

Purchase and Use ONLY White Hair Care Products! The 24 Month-Hair-Growth Timetable:

You need a Moisturizing Program for Reversing Extraordinarily Dry, Brittle Hair, and when it comes to selecting your Conditioning and Shampoo Hair Care Products, don't ever use **Black Hair Products.** Use **ONLY shampoo and conditioner that are White Hair Care Products**. As I've mentioned before, I think those **from Nexxus Products are best.**

If a **Chemical No-LYE Relaxer Kit** has been applied to your hair, or if you have **Self-Applied** and **COMBED** this chemical through your hair, you can correct over 90 percent of the problems by using **ONLY Humectress Moisturizing Conditioner** with **Therappe Shampoo. (Both are from NEXXUS.)**

A ShamBOOsie Tip: Please don't go out and purchase just ONE of the products on the list to see if it will work because it Will Not WORK! Either follow the plan or DON'T! It will only cost you about $35.00 to learn how amazing every product really is. Purchase and use **Crème Press Hairdressing from Dudley Products.** A Weekly Treatment program is every three, four, or five days, until the damage and the exceptional dryness are brought under control. You will know when the weekly treatment program has WORKED because your hair will be so soft to the touch and the breakage will be brought to an end. Then your weekly treatment program is every five days.

The Roller Setting:
ShamBOOsie Suggests You Set Your Hair Now and Then

This is a wonderful way to give your hair a rest from the use of a ceramic flat iron, curling iron, and blow dryers. When you add a nickel-size dollop of **PCA Moisture Retainer** from **Dudley's Products** to about six to eight ounces of **Fantastic Body Setting Lotion,** then spray it into the hair just before putting the hair on rollers; the comb out will be **so soft to touch,** bouncy and full of body. The hair of the woman of color is seldom **soft to the touch,** bouncy, and full of body. Setting the hair on rollers every now and then is very good for the hair.

You MUST still add just a light film of **Crème Press Hairdressing** throughout the hair to help keep it **so soft to the touch.** As you recall, **Crème Press Hairdressing** keeps the hair strong and **so soft to the touch all day, every day.** Just be sure not to overdo it or apply the product on just one part of the hair. One more thing, use a Blow Dryer and a brush to remove just a portion of the curls or set the hair on large rollers. Set the rollers in an un-exact pattern and use a large-tooth comb to comb the hair in the opposite way to which it was rolled. Then finish the style using your fingers. The complete list of products you should have on hand at all times can be found below.

Dudley's Products

I spent many years very early in my career getting it right with my clients' hair; it was the most important thing. So I went searching for all of the answers. I wanted to know what were the best Conditioners and how each of them worked, if they worked at all. I bought all kinds of different bottles and jars of stuff and tried them on my Clients' hair to see how they made their hair feel, look, and if they stopped breakage. I refuse to use a single hair product on my customers that doesn't deliver. So what is found here are some of the best products available in the business, and you can totally trust every one of them. I want your hair to be "Pretty Hair" healthy hair, no matter how long or short you want it to be. And that goes for your baby girl's hair, too.

When Hair Was Relaxed with a "Conditioning LYE Relaxer"

- **Deluxe Shampoo**
- **Hair Rebuilder Penetrating Conditioner**: Leave in for twenty minutes while wearing a plastic cap. Add two dime-size dollops of PCA Moisture Retainer to six ounces of Fantastic Body Setting Lotion before Detangling Wet Hair and for SOFTER Bouncy Hair with Body.
- **Crème Press Hairdressing and Pressing Crème**
- Never flat iron or Curl the Hair without applying **Crème Press;** use **lightly** on every strand of the hair before using a flat iron or curling iron.

For Roller Sets

- **Purchase and use ShamBOOsie's Favorites for the Finished Look**
- **Deluxe Shampoo**
- Fantastic Body Setting Lotion for Detangling Wet Hair
- PCA Moisture Retainer - add a two dime-size dollops to six ounces of Fantastic Body Setting Lotion.
- **Crème Press Hairdressing and Pressing Crème**
- Total Control Styling Spray

ShamBOOsie's Favorite OIL for Basing the Scalp before Applying Chemical Relaxer

- Vitamin AD&E Hair and SCALP Conditioner

The Best for Dandruff Treatment:

- Dudley's Dandruff Shampoo
- Hair Rebuilder Penetrating Conditioner
- Fantastic Body Setting Lotion
- Panthenol Leave-in Conditioner

Hair Care Products
What they Can and Cannot Do

One of my main reasons for writing books about Hair Care is my sincere desire to help you understand why you continue to have serious problems with your hair. I'd like to help you solve those problems, if possible, and teach you how to grow your hair as long and as healthy as possible. The discoveries outlined in this book will bring an end to more than 250 years of the black woman's inability to grow and keep her hair long, flowing, and healthy. I believe that greater than 95 percent of all black women can grow a Pretty head of hair with ease. Simply follow the rules and stick to my plan!

Beautiful Black Hair

Things go wrong when the rules of proper Hair Care are broken and most women break all of the rules all the time. This includes chemical applications, where the worst mistakes are made, and the misuse and use of inferior hair products. The biggest problem area and the cause of the majority of the problems involve the use of products not suitable for the overall health and GROWTH of your hair. Use of shoddy, ineffective hair products is responsible for your hair problems.

ShamBOOsie's Hair Wellness Approach to Hair Growth is designed to fulfill the needs of your hair by making it possible to GROW a beautiful healthy mane with ease. A woman's hair should be **so soft to the touch,** healthy, and strong. Don't you feel beautiful, special, and really good about yourself when your hair looks good?

For years women of color have had problems keeping their hair on the heads long enough for it to GROW long, flowing hair. Healthy hair is your goal, even if you don't want your hair to be long or chemically relaxed, and **ShamBOOsie's Hair Wellness Approach to Hair GROWTH** is about helping you **Have it your way.** Getting their hair to grow healthy is what it's all about!

The important question is *how can black women Chemically Relax their hair every six, seven, or eight weeks for the rest of their lives and keep the hair Healthy, Strong, Soft, Pretty, and on their heads?* Until now, this question remained unanswered. If you are desperately searching for a way to get your hair to grow, **ShamBOOsie's Hair Wellness Approach to Hair GROWTH** will end that search once and for all.

Stop Relaxing at Home!

The first change to make is to stop combing relaxer through your own hair and the hair of your daughters. Although this book and the companion DVD illustrate the proper application technique for chemical relaxer, I DO NOT recommend you do the relaxer service at home. A salon professional should handle all chemical services such as applying Permanent Hair Color, Relaxers, Curls, and Highlights. The step-by-step guides that come with this System are provided so that you will know if the services being rendered are done properly. An educated client is always best.

ShamBOOsie has created a revolutionary Chemical Relaxer Application System. You must discover and master the application of the **Conditioning Lye Relaxer, which is** an extraordinary Conditioning LYE Relaxer System that will be discussed in more detail later. This is an **EXACT** Relaxer System that requires the **EXACT** application method to achieve the **EXACT** results and GROWTH. The results will be remarkable. **ShamBOOsie's Hair Wellness Approach to Hair Growth** offers a complete line of Superior Hair Care Products that are unrivaled by anything before their time and that can be found on store shelves all over the country.

Taking Care of Your Hair: The Basics

My purpose is to share with you the exact ways of servicing your hair from start to finish. Often you expect the Low-End Hair products you use to do more than the job they were designed for. For example, many of you think the use of grease and oil is the answer for everything that is wrong with your hair. **There is NEVER a reason to put grease and heavy oil on your hair!** You blame the products for dryness, breakage, the hair's inability to hold curl, lack of shine, and its inability to relax properly and GROW, but all while you're GROWING new hair. Seldom do you blame yourself, the one really responsible for your hair problems. The products you've been using are largely responsible for your hair loss, and you either put them on your hair or allowed someone else to put them on your hair.

113

A ShamBOOsie Need-to-Know Tip: Cosmetology and The Study of Hair are EXACT sciences, and Quality Hair Care Products are made according to those sciences. If you select your Hair Care Products that are High-End, especially Moisturizing Conditioners and Shampoos, then use them often; they will scientifically produce the results they were created to deliver. There is never a reason for guessing, which is exactly what most people do, even Hairstylists. There are EXACT rules, methods, concepts, and ways to do whatever you need to do to your hair. You don't have to guess how to use a Chemical Relaxer, Permanent Hair Color, or which Relaxer is the right one for your hair.

There is no guessing as to how to give your hair the perfect haircut because there are EXACT ways to cut every hairstyle. You shouldn't have to guess about the best shampoo, conditioner, setting lotion, setting gel, Chemical Relaxer, or even who is the best person to style and service your hair. You don't have to guess how long to leave color on, if you should bleach your hair, or how to mix setting lotion.

Hair Care 101

What is meant by the phrase retouch of the relaxer? A Retouch, Retrace, and Touch-up are all same thing. All three must be performed correctly and will destroy your hair if misunderstood or misapplied. If you don't believe me, peep in the mirror at your hair for just ten seconds. The fact of the matter is about 100,000 Hairdressers and most of the 20 million black women across the country do not fully understand what is meant by Retouch, Retrace, or Touch-up. The prefix *re* means once more, afresh, or anew but in the context of hair care it doesn't mean to the same hair! Retouch applies to the new growth only!

Most women think the hair reverts and has to be relaxed over and over. If this is the case, you get to re-relax your hair hoping to straighten your hair about six to eight times each year. If you add up the danger of relaxing your own hair over and over, the use of a No-Lye home relaxer kit, and the fact that you are combing the chemical through the hair over and over, there is almost a 100 percent guarantee that you will lose most, if not all, of your hair. Does losing all of your hair and being bald ring a very loud bell? Once the damage is done, you can't unring the bell! There isn't really such a thing as **Black Hair Care Products or White Hair Care Products,** although I will be using such terms when referring to products many times in this book. You are more familiar with the words **Black Hair Care Products.**

True Story: I Can GROW My Hair All the Way to the Floor!

Keep in mind that if you were to MASTER the use of Conditioners, it would change your entire life. My Doctor is woman from India. She is my primary care Doctor at the VA Hospital. Last week she learned that I wrote Hair Care books, for women of color. It wasn't long before we were talking about the hair women of color use for their weaves. My doctor said that in India, the longer a woman grows her hair, the more beautiful she is considered to be. **She said, "I can GROW my hair all the way to the floor!"** Then she told me that she was having a problem finding a shampoo she could use and that every one she tried caused a skin irritation. Her problem is the fragrances manufacturers put in their shampoos to make them smell good.

So I am in search of a Green High-End Shampoo that will not cause skin irritation. If it's true that there is such a thing as **Black Hair Care Products and White Hair Care Products,** I will have to find **my Doctor a line of Indian Hair Care Products.** No product manufacturers have the ability to make Hair Care Products according to ethnicity. They are *HAIR* Care Products that are made for HAIR. There are

115

Beautiful Black Hair

High-End, Quality Hair Care Products that will work very well and there are low-end, poor quality Hair Care Products that don't work at all.

Your Conditioner Selections

The job of your main conditioner is to Treat, Soften, and Strengthen your hair, and even that job will vary with different types of Conditioners. The Conditioner is the "Real Muscle" that makes and keeps the Cuticle or outer layer of each hair strand smooth, resilient, and as healthy as possible. The conditioner will also feed the hair and fill it with many wonderful natural properties. It can make your hair strong, bouncy, shiny, and soft all at once.

See the chapter **on Conditioners and Treatments**

The Bonds of the Hair: Just the Basics

The bonds are identical in all hair. Not only is the growth of your hair Mother Nature's business, the makeup of hair is also her business. The major types of bonds are the S for sulfur bonds, H for hydrogen bonds, D for disulfide bonds, and P for peptide bonds, all of which are natural chemical bonds. They all fall under the heading of protein. Everything on the earth that has life is made of protein. God created all life from the earth. "Now the Lord God had formed out of the ground all the beasts of the field and all the birds of the air" (Genesis 2:19 NIV).

As you can see, we and every other living thing are all made from the same stuff of the earth. It is no wonder that protein is such a vital part of our makeup. So protein becomes a major key to keeping the hair strong, stopping breakage, keeping the hair on the head, and GROWING longer, healthier, and more beautiful than ever. The quality, quantity, and type of protein are also very important. So don't

116

go out and buy a Concentrated Protein Conditioner and put it on your hair, hoping to STOP your hair breakage. If there is a No-LYE Relaxer Kit in your hair, a Concentrated Protein Conditioner would cause your head to become as BALD as a baby's bottom. You need not be concerned about any of this. **ShamBOOsie's Hair Wellness Approach to Hair Growth** has taken care of everything for you. Just follow the plan, and it will deliver.

The bonds determine the shape and strength of the hair, as well as its ability to become weak and if the cuticle layer will become damaged easily. The healthier, softer, and stronger we keep the cuticle or outer layer of the hair, the better chance it will have to GROW longer. The bonds determine if the hair will be soft, wiry, resistant, or porous, which mean its ability to retain SOFTNESS. The bonds also determine the structure of the hair, the elasticity of the hair, which means its ability to stretch, retract, and bend easily.

The bonds determine if hair will be curly, wavy, or straight; they give the hair its natural curls. If the hair is naturally straight, the bonds determine if the hair can be chemically altered to become curly, and how well it would hold its new curls. The natural bonds of the hair establish all of these factors and many others. (Just thought you needed to know.) One more thing, the beauty giant L'Oreal Paris, which owns and manufacturers most of the black brands of Chemical No-LYE Relaxer Kits, will leave you believing that black women have dry skin, dry hair, and no shine on the hair.

Special Effects

Each individual Quality Hair Care Product in **ShamBOOsie's Hair Wellness Approach to Hair Growth** has special properties that are designed to positively affect one or more of the natural bonds of the hair. When you apply each product as instructed, which is just

117

that simple, it will have the EXACT effect on those bonds that it was designed to have, and the desired results will occur every time. If you try to save money by using a cheap substitute for even one of the four Conditioner Products in the program, it will change the results dramatically and the outcome cannot be as predicted. If you are going to do this, close the book, and get on with doing things your way. I wish you luck!

A ShamBOOsie Tip: The hair should never be preshampooed the day it is to be chemically relaxed or thirty-six hours before. The cleansing of the hair must take place during the chemical process. If you shampoo, get caught in the rain, go swimming, or wet the hair in any way and then attempt to dry the hair and get a LYE Relaxer the same day, your entire scalp would be "on fire" in less than five minutes. For this reason you must always tell your Salon Professional if you have wet your hair within the past forty-eight hours before getting a relaxer.

There is Necessary Water and Unnecessary Water

Water used to dilute conditioners; mixed with temporary color or setting lotion; used in a spray bottle; used for rinsing curly perms, bleach, unwanted color, and dirt; used in shampooing; and used to rinse Neutralizing Shampoo and residuals from conditioners is necessary. Then there is unnecessary water like a rainy day, a humid day, sweating after two hours of exercising, water from a water fight with the kids, and the one type of water that is most dangerous for your hair—dripping water from the rinse after the removal of color, perm, bleach, and shampooing before applying a Neutralizing Shampoo and before applying your conditioners.

Water Dilutes and Weakens Product

Water is used to dilute concentrated formulas but here is a warning, when water is mixed with Neutralizing Shampoo, it weakens the

Neutralizer in the shampoo causing it to become less effective. It is so important to towel blot or soak up excess water that is dripping from the hair after each rinse. When it comes to the chemical relaxer, water will remove the content of the product itself from the hair, but it will *NOT* alter the strength of the chemical or its effect of eating through the hair.

In short, the Neutralizer, which is in shampoo form, will stop the Chemical from straightening your hair. If you don't STOP the action of the Chemical, it will STOP on its own, hours after you leave the Salon. By that time the Chemical will have eaten through your hair. Watered down, weakened Neutralizer Shampoo will not properly STOP the Chemical from working. It must be full strength inside the thick shampoo lather.

Holding Agents

The job of the setting lotion is to soften the cuticle layer so that it will comb easier. It also acts as an artificial bond to help the hair hold its curl from a wet set or when the hair is blown into style with a blow dryer and brush. This set will last two to three days depending on the condition, strength, and texture of the hair. If your hair is to ever hold a curl after it has been relaxed, you will need an artificial bonding product, a holding agent such as setting gel, hair spray, spritz, mousse or setting lotion, and a hot curling iron.

Styling Sprays should never be used without Crème Press Hairdressing! The sprays will dry out the hair. **Crème Press Hairdressing by Dudley Products** is the best I have ever used, and I have used many brands and types of hairdressing. **Crème Press Hairdressing** keeps the hair soft, cancels the dryness from the spray, and gives the hair a brilliant shine. The curls will hold all day long; when using hairdressing, remember **A Little Dab Will Do Ya!** Use in dime-size portions, and as

119

much as you need to cover every hair strand. **ShamBOOsie doesn't use OIL on any Client's hair—ever!**

A Hairdressing Tip

Protection, protection, protection is essential—you must remember this. Crème Press Hairdressing by Dudley Products is the one product you should have more of on hand than any other, except conditioner. I can't began to tell you how extremely important it is to use this product during every dry set, wet set, after blow drying the hair, and before hot curling. This product is a must. Crème Press Hairdressing will protect the hair from hot irons and will offset any and all dryness caused by whatever else you have used before dressing the hair. If you have Crème Press, you should not have dry or brittle hair.

A Very Important Tip

The moisture from each of the products you use will add varying degrees of SOFTNESS. However, they do not add enough moisture/softness to protect the hair against the Dryness that will occur after the hair is blown dry, after a Wet Set, after drying under a Hood Dryer, after Hot Curling, or after the use of a flat iron. This is normal, so relax. What is not normal is the Exceptional, Extraordinary Dryness that will always occur from combing a Chemical No-LYE Relaxer Kit through the hair.

A more Concentrated Moisture Retainer, such as **Crème Press Hairdressing**, will be needed to maintain the hair's softness after it has been serviced and styled. I highly recommend this very important cream hairdressing, which must be applied lightly (in dime-size portions) daily to keep moisture and softness in your hair. It will not interfere with the hair's ability to hold curl, if anything it will enhance it. Recently I was made aware of a New Concentrated Moisturizing Conditioner from Nexxus Products. It's a new Concentrated Moisturizing Deep Conditioning Treatment, a sister to Humectress Moisturizing Conditioner on store shelves across the country.

Chapter 7

Easy Combing for Baby Girl

ShamBOOsie's Texture Waving to Loosen the Natural Curls

Guaranteed: No Scalp Burns Ever and No Guesswork!

Mothers are Mothers Because It Was God's Plan

You must agree that black mothers are by far the most amazing, most wonderful, most beautiful creatures God ever created. After he created the universe and the earth in six days, and man, he saved the very best of all his creations for last. Then God created woman. She was to be mother of every man, woman, and child. She is in constant contact with her maker for he holds her high. She is my princess, my Beautiful Queen, and Pillar of strength, and because she is a mother or capable of being a mother, no man is stronger. Yet she is as delicate as a rose and should be held gently. She is a loving woman and my best friend. She is emotionally sensitive, and if not careful, one could easily break her heart. She should be given every opportunity to change her mind about anything and everything, without notice, and she takes the opportunity, given or not. She is a woman.

Beautiful Black Hair

The black woman is as bright in color as a morning sun. She is yellow, red, brown, and as dark as the twilight of an evening sunset and midnight—black, beautifully black. She is a mixture of as many skin colors and textures of hair, as there are women on the planet. This black woman is a mixture of every race of people from every corner of the world. Her eyes are blue, brown, green, hazel, grayish tan, and as black as onyx. She is a shapely, with hips and full lips and incredible cheekbone. She has a smile to die for, and is a most beautiful sight to see. She has style, the most rhythm, a laugh, a cry, and a smile all of her very own. She is a black woman, and the mother of the entire human family.

She is sexy, sensuous, and soft to the touch and so much more. Because she is the maker of every man, she is the most beautiful, most marvelous, and miraculous part of who I am. When she stands next to me, I feel stronger, taller, and the most man I can ever be; every time I am given the opportunity to hold her and love her, it is an event and occasion during which something wonderful happens. She should be graciously loved, pampered, caressed, cared for, made to feel safe, and given gifts and roses often just because. She is a black woman, the mother of life and living. She is completely woman, in every sense of the word—special, unique and lovely in all her lovely ways. It is my privilege to do all that I can as a man of beautiful artistry, to enhance such beauty, that of a black woman.

Little Girls are Gifts from the Creator

My precious little darlings—three daughters, six granddaughters, and five great-granddaughters—are the very beat of my heart. They are gifts from the Creator and not guests but authorities in their homes. By that I mean that they are most important, and all my living revolves around them. The day they arrived, they took over the lives of everyone in the home, and that's the way it should be.

I realize that you mothers are sensitive to the many different cries of your baby. Everything that comes in contact with your baby becomes hers alone. She has her own clothing, bathing products, bottles and nipples, towels, and washcloths. She has her own bedding, feeding utensils, food, shampoos, hairbrushes, and combs. You wash her clothing separately with washing products designed especially for her, and you store all of her things in a place that is "just for her."

Mommy It Hurts So Bad: The Cry of a Little Girl

The hair care process that is commonly referred to as "having your hair done" can really be a traumatic ordeal for **black girls.** You don't want things to be this way, so let's find another way. It can be heart wrenching for mothers, too. In some cases, this experience can be so upsetting that it can leave emotional scars. Because of their hair's coarse and sometimes thick texture, the child's hair is difficult to comb. Can you imagine what it is like when a child has to endure the painful pulling and tugging when Mommy tries to comb her hair? Surely most black women can relate to this because they can recall their own childhood memories of this ordeal.

Sometimes a child will ask why it hurts so badly, and the child may think that Mommy is angry with her. At this point, Mom doesn't know what to say, but she certainly wishes there was a better way.

Take More Time and Slow the Process Way Down

- Shampoo and then condition her hair with Humectress Moisturizing Conditioner to help soften her hair, and towel dry the hair.
- Separate the hair into as many small sections as you need the hair to be in to style it. To make combing her hair easier and less painful, hold each section firmly with the thumb and the fingers

125

with one hand. The idea is to keep the hair from being pulled at the scalp. If you hold the hair firmly with your finger and thumb you will only pull on the hair from the ends to where it is being held with your fingers. As you detangle each section move the fingers closer and closer toward the scalp until each section of the hair is detangled.

Baby GIRL
ShamBOOsie's Beautiful Brown Lady Babies

As I mentioned, I have three daughters, six granddaughters, and five great-granddaughters. For these fourteen Beautiful Brown Baby Girls to have their hair relaxed in a salon every six to eight weeks (at $50 each) would cost approximately $700.00, and poor families cannot handle that cost. So they choose what I call a Trick in a Box—the No-Lye Relaxer Kit. It seems like a great idea and it only costs ten dollars, but then reality checks in! **I have written this hair care book to correct this problem and to teach every black mother and female to master the art of applying the Chemical LYE Relaxer!** You should know ShamBOOsie would never use a No-Lye Relaxer Box Kit on anyone's hair—ever!

Little black girls are not born with straight hair; in fact it's just the opposite. Their mothers begin at a very young age trying to give their hair a smooth look around the face and as a result, causing damage from which the hair will never recover. Today some moms will bring a Chemical Relaxer into the picture for girls as young as two years old. The problem with this is that the Chemical and their lack of knowledge of what they are doing will destroy their daughter's hair.

I am so tired of seeing the harm and the hurt these Chemicals are causing in the little hearts of our Beautiful Brown Baby Girls! Their mothers cannot possibly explain why this is happening to their daughters' hair. Pictures of the chemically damaged hair of little black girls are frozen in my memory. It is still very difficult for me to see ShamBOOsie's Beautiful Brown Baby Girls whose mothers have done what they thought would make combing their daughters' hair easier but ended up destroying their hair instead.

These Chemical No-Lye Relaxer Kits are taking every bit of their hair OUT! The most obvious FIX is to teach black mothers how to properly relax their daughters' hair using a Conditioning LYE Relaxer, with NO Scalp Burns EVER! Then teach them how to Shampoo and Condition their hair, and how to select the best High-End Hair Care Products so that their hair will GROW right down their backs!

Chemicals and Little Girls' Hair

You MUST Master the Art of Applying the Chemical LYE Relaxer!
Today mothers are resorting to Chemical Relaxers very early in their little girls' lives in hopes of alleviating a rather painful daily hair ritual of having to comb their little girls' hair because it is a dreadful experience for their daughters. But the Chemicals are not getting the job done. There are chemical burns to the scalp, their little girl's hair becomes extremely dry, it pops and breaks constantly, and there are many other Hair Care issues. During the first eighteen years of her life, she will GROW and lose all of her hair dozens of times, but it will only happen because of mistakes the mom will make along the way.

The worst mistake is purchasing the no-lye relaxer kit because the makers imply that the product is safe to use. Instead it is the most destructive Chemical on the market. This Chemical will destroy your child's hair. The idea is to learn how to care for her hair, and please know that it's very much the same as caring for your own hair. Just about everything is the same. It doesn't matter that she's a little girl.

After the age of tw0, Hair Care Products aren't made for the age of people; they're all made for hair.

For a black female child, having her hair combed daily is more painful than one can imagine. She cries many times throughout the entire process. She MUST have the hair combed every day for the first ten to twelve years of her life and mostly without having it chemically relaxed. So many mothers are chemically relaxing the little girl's hair to make the process easier for both the mother and the daughter. The only problem I have with it is that mothers won't learn how to use the chemical relaxer properly.

If you are going to have your daughter's the hair relaxed, or if you are going to do it yourself, then you must commit to caring for it, or she will lose most, if not all, of it. Use this book to learn how to relax her hair and don't take any short cuts during the process. If you can manage to wait until she is twelve years old for the chemical relaxer, the child will be able to care for her own hair. Commit now to purchasing the High-End products this book recommends because nothing else will work to take the best care of her hair and yours. The two of you can use the same products. But the reality is that she MUST deal with this impossible hair from age two and throughout her entire life. It is time for someone to bring an end to the struggle.

Every time the hair is chemically relaxed, in just six to eight weeks the new GROWTH of one-quarter to one-half inch returns and the process MUST occur again and again. The process must continue or she will lose the hair that has been relaxed. Here is another very good reason why you should learn how to handle this chemical. The very health and GROWTH of her hair will depend on it. It is this fact that supports the factual finding that women of color will collectively spend billions of dollars every year trying to find SOLUTIONS to so many hair care issues.

At the end of each year they have very little hair to show for the enormous amount of money they have spent. The only way to change this is to learn how to do things the right way. We have created those SOLUTIONS; we have found the ways to make it all work.

The Toolbox: Here is What You Need

- Blow Dryer
- Comb Attachment – Willie Morrow
- A Champion #99 Shampoo Rake Comb
- Champion Tuff Comb 8" #28
- Twelve 8" Black Tail Comb Combs #263
- If you can't find Champion combs, Ace Combs are a good replacement
- Cushion Brush and Vent Brush
- **There is a comb attachment for your hair dryer, and you can find it online. It's made by Willie Morrow, and it's called the Solano Willie Morrow Blow Dry Nozzle. Find it online by typing keywords:** Solano Willie Morrow Blow Dry Nozzle. I have one that I have had for over twenty years. It is made of heavy-duty plastic and will last a lifetime. When you dry her hair or yours, this comb attachment will allow you to remove over 80 percent of the natural curl from the hair.
- **You want to purchase a Champion hard rubber *#99 Rake Comb*, which will cost between, $7 and $10.00 at your local beauty supply store. This comb will last her lifetime.** Ask for the comb by its brand name, **Champion.** You will see cheaper combs that will look the same, but Champion combs are the best hard rubber combs. There are other hard rubber Rake Combs on the market, which are okay if you can't find a Champion. This is the perfect

comb for the baby's hair and your hair also. It is very strong and will last for years. This comb will make combing your daughter's hair much easier and much less painful.

- You can apply Crème Press Hairdressing to every strand of the hair while the hair is still damp. It will slow the drying process down because the hairdressing will interfere because of the moisture content. Or you may apply a little Crème Press after each section of the hair is dried. This will be the perfect opportunity to use a flat iron to smooth the hair even more. This process will be the same with or without chemicals in the hair. The Crème Press will leave the hair silky soft and with a lot of sheen.

- I used to watch my sister Denise attempting to comb her daughter's hair, which was extremely long, thick, kinky, and very dry. Her daughter was having a very unpleasant experience, and from the look on her mother's face, she hated the ordeal just as much as her daughter. Her daughter would be in tears because her mother would place the comb in the hair and just pull on it. I couldn't offer any advice because I didn't know anything about hair care back then.

- Each day of the week, if you will apply the Crème Press Hairdressing lightly to every strand of her hair, the hair will become softer and easier to comb each day. Don't concern yourself with trying to keep the hair straight around the face and hairline. Allow the hair around the face to be as natural looking as it is. Even if you were to get it smooth around the face, it will be natural looking in about one hour after you finish with her hair. Pulling the hair back tightly will damage the hair follicles around the face and cause baldness.

ShamBOOsie's Texture Waving Application is about relieving her dreadful pain, for as long as she lives. and I am sorry, I wouldn't wish what she must endure for a lifetime on anyone. I can do all

I can to make living with overly curly hair a lot easier, which what Easy Curling is all about. First remember never shampoo her hair before applying chemical relaxer. The scalp becomes very sensitive and will burn within five minutes of applying the chemicals. Always allow about four days between shampooing and getting the retouch, relaxer, or **ShamBOOsie's Texture Waving** application. The hair will become clean by the end of the process. **It is very important NOT to use a box kit or a No-Lye Relaxer.**

The **Conditioning LYE Relaxer** is much better. If you have used a No-Lye Relaxer in her hair, the chemical LYE Relaxer will have little or no effect on her hair because the No-Lye Relaxer neutralizes the bonds of the hair the first time around. Remember, **ShamBOOsie's Texture Wave** is simply a Chemical LYE Relaxer, and when this chemical is left on the hair too long, say fifteen to eighteen minutes, it will straighten the hair. With each RETOUCH the chemical MUST be applied to the NEW GRORTH ONLY. **ShamBOOsie's Texture Waves** are very difficult to do over and over again because each time the chemical is applied to the hair it will relax the hair a little straighter.

A Chemical Tip:

With **ShamBOOsie's Texture Waving**, the Chemical LYE Relaxer has to be applied quickly. To apply **ShamBOOsie's Texture Wave** to the hair, the first application is different from the normal Relaxer Retouch Application. It MUST be a LYE Relaxer. The Chemical needs to get on ALL the hair in one or two minutes, so apply the chemical with the fingers. The retouch application is very different! The chemical is applied ONLY to the new growth, but it, too, must be applied quickly. The person applying the product cannot do any talking while working because this will slow down the application process. And sometimes, one minute longer can be too long. When you do your own **Texture Waving** you are forced to comb the chemical through hair that has already been treated with the relaxer.

The art of **chemically texture waving** overly curly hair involves knowing a few secrets about the way the chemical works, the chemical's effect on the hair, and what actually takes place throughout the process. All the bonds in the hair that cause the hair to be overly curly will be altered and gone forever. The secret is to not destroy all the natural bonds and leave about 30 percent of the natural curl in the hair. This is why if the chemical is left on the hair too long it will straighten the hair, and the hair will not revert. It takes between twelve to fifteen minutes for hair to totally relax straight; starting from the time the chemical first comes in contact with the first section of the hair.

With the rinsing process, the chemical should be totally removed from the hair in about one or two minutes. This process works best when it takes place in a salon. It's a guessing game and something could go wrong at any time, meaning you straighten the hair, so keep your eyes on the work and the clock. Everyone's hair will react differently depending on the texture and strength of the hair.

This Is Very Important!
The entire scalp and a full inch around the hairline and the ears MUST be covered with an oil-based grease! A tingling sensation will occur in the area of the first section where the application began. At this point, you will have approximately two to five minutes to complete the process.

If You Decide to Chemically Relax Her Yourself
Remember that when you start the process of relaxing her hair or yours, even if that is a **ShamBOOsie's Texture Wave** it will be very difficult to stop using the chemical without losing the hair. The use of

quality Conditioners will be her greatest benefactor. The hair has to be retouched on time, every six to eight weeks, so chose one: six, seven, or eight. Retouch the hair every six weeks if the hair GROWS fast and every seven or eight weeks if the hair GROWS slowly. Just don't skip around, every six weeks or every seven weeks or every eight weeks. At nine or ten years of age, your daughter should have enough experience to do the needed Conditioners and shampoos, every four or five days. If she is younger, you will have to do the Conditioning treatment.

I had a conversation with my oldest daughter the other day. She told me that my nine-year-old granddaughter, Miranda, wants a relaxer put in her hair. I told my daughter to make sure that the Chemical is a Conditioning LYE Relaxer and NEVER a No-Lye Relaxer Kit. The hair, even if there are no chemicals in it, MUST BE SHAMPOOED AND CONDITIONED every five days, like clockwork, with the proper products. If you intend to do this at home, follow these guidelines: **Follow the Plan** "A Healthier, Safer, More Comfortable Way to Relax Hair." Use a *Regular Conditioning Lye Relaxer*. But make sure you have used my relaxer application technique several times in practice before you try this on your daughter's hair.

You do not want to get the hair bone *straight* when she's between the age of two and twelve years old, and NEVER Comb the chemical through her hair with a fine-tooth comb. You only want to *loosen the curls* removing about 30 percent of the curl. To do this you have to get the chemical on and off the hair in about ten minutes. Start the timing after the chemical has been applied to all of the hair. Use your hands to do the application.

1. If the child is small, prepare the counter top next to the kitchen sink by padding it with a blanket. This is going to be tedious work, and you want to do all you can to protect her eyes.

2. When the hair is ready to rinse, quickly place the child on her back on top of the padded counter.

3. Put earplugs in her ears to keep out the water and residue from the chemical.

4. Make sure she keeps her eyes closed. Place a small towel over her eyes and have her hold it in place with both hands.

5. If she is old enough, use the complete system of application in the chapter on **A Healthier, Safer, More Comfortable Way to Relax Hair.**

6. Make sure the water temperature is warm and perfect for her.

7. While you support her head over the sink, remove the chemical entirely from the hair according to the sections that were applied first or according the instructions in the chapter on relaxer application.

8. Remember, it is not necessary to get the hair completely straight. It is actually better to leave some curl in the hair. Bone straight is never a good idea. Even the slightest wave in the hair will indicate that there is still some life left in the hair. The natural curl is the life in your hair and removing all of it leaves the hair without body.

9. Remember also that the hair will get even straighter during the retouch applications. There will be many of them, one every eight weeks or six times a year.

Some Styling Ideas for Children

Use a flat iron to smooth out the hair. Braids are good but make sure they're not too tight. Spiral curls, plaits, bangs, ponytails, and braided ponytails are appropriate styles for girls. If your daughter's hair is very short, wearing the hair natural is an option, and all the same products can be used. Ribbons, barrettes, bows, headbands, and many other hair ornaments are available.

As a black woman, your beauty is not lessened by the appearance of your kinky hair; instead your hair identifies you as beautiful and black. It is like all of the other pleasing and attractive qualities you have. There are women of other races and nationalities that would give anything to have some of the physical characteristics that black women are known to possess. I get to work with some very beautiful black women.

No matter how much time you put into combing, pulling, pressing, chemically relaxing, and smoothing the hair around your face, and throughout your head, in six to eight weeks, those kinky little beauties return. Those pretty little kinky, curly, nappy strands around the face will return every time for the rest of your life, just as they have for as long as you have been alive.

Very tight braiding will pull out a lot of hair. It must be done with much less tension. These are tiny strands, and they break easily. It's easy to pull them out from the roots and kill the follicles, preventing GROWTH in those areas. Do everything you can to ease the strain on the finer hair around the face and in the temple areas. Gently comb her hair around her face forward and allow it to be natural. Natural is beautiful. It is what it is. The solution is simple: open your eyes and see the hair of your little black girl, which is lovely and even fascinatingly beautiful. Know that no matter what it is, it's an important part of her overall beauty.

A Gentle Touch: She Loves It!

I get a lot of e-mail from mothers, and I am amazed by some of the things mothers are doing to their daughters' hair. One mother wrote me about her eighteen-month-old daughter. She had been entering her baby in beauty contests and evidently it had made her some money. The problem was that the baby's hair fell out, which is normal for eighteen-month-olds. The mother wanted to know what I'd recommend to get the baby's hair to grow back, and like many of the women that write asking the same thing about their hair, she wanted the growth to happen immediately.

The thing that bothered me most was that the mother said she was considering having someone put a weave in the eighteen-month-old baby's hair. I wrote back and told the mother that she should be ashamed of herself and to leave her baby's hair alone. Do you think there's a hairdresser somewhere out there that would put a weave in this eighteen-month-old baby's hair? You better believe it! They will do anything for money.

So, what about your little girl's hair? How should you care for it? Keep it as simple as possible, and don't be overly concerned about it. Tell her that her hair is pretty often. Baby girls can be born with a head full of hair or they can be as bald headed as ShamBOOsie. Sometimes boys are born with more hair than girls, and the hair of babies is many times as fragile as they are. Everything about them is constantly growing and growing back again and again. Their hair could fall out, leaving their scalp clean in places on the head for months before returning; that's just the nature of things. Just treat your baby girl's hair the same way you treat the rest of her. Don't be overly concerned about the fall out; the hair will GROW back.

It's very much like her teeth; they will fall out and grow back. Lots of things like lint will cling to her hair, so you have to keep it clean and put pretty things in it, I suggest ribbons but not if she can put them in her mouth. She's the baby, so try to be as gentle with her hair as you are with the rest of her. Use special shampoos for babies with beautiful fragrances that will leave her hair and skin feeling soft to the touch and smelling good. Wash her face and hands once or twice a day or more if you choose, with a warm soft cloth but no soap just warm clean water. Keep her tiny belly button as clean as possible, and always using the gentle loving touches that she loves! Be her mother naturally; it will be a very natural thing for you to handle. You are her mother.

Read books about babies and how to care for them, it's already been done many times. Buy teaching DVD's to teach them how to read and let them watch TV and learn. Before drawing her bath, place one of her large towels in the bottom of her bath basin to add a little cushion. You should always look for the softest towels, sponges, and washcloths you can find. When bathing her, **never leave her alone in her bath to talk on the telephone, answer the door, or for any reason.** It makes better sense to wrap her in a towel and take her with you. Just as you test her milk and formulas to make sure they are not too cool or too hot, make sure her bath water is the perfect temperature.

So How Should You Care for Your Daughter's Hair?

At about age two her hair will probably go through a metamorphosis. The thing to remember is that a baby's hair is in *perfect condition* from birth until about age two. The products you use should be very gentle, such as a "no tears" shampoo with rich lather that will clean her hair without skin irritation. Use shampoos with good-smelling fragrances, those that will leave her hair and skin feeling soft to the touch. The baby's hair will get tangled now and then, so use a gentle, detangling shampoo that will make her hair pretty, silky, soft, and more manageable. Hold the sections of hair between the thumb and four fingers, while you comb the ends, this will keep you from pulling on her hair and causing her pain.

Beautiful Black Hair

There are a few things mothers must keep in mind when dealing with their daughter's hair. You were once her age. Your mother had to comb your hair every day, and you dreaded it as much as your daughter does now. You recall the PAIN! One of the biggest problems is finding the right COMBS and other tools you will be using to manage her hair with and the products. Her hair needs the very same conditioners and shampoos you would use on your hair. After her "baby years" are over, her hair becomes a horrific challenge as it was for you.

It seems you would want to find a way to handle her hair so that it will be much easier and less painful for her. That's what this section of the book aims to accomplish. I simply want to offer a few suggestions to help you soften the many episodes of having to wake up every day and put your daughter through the drudgery of having her hair combed.

Managing Black Hair Can Be Difficult without Understanding!

Most often a little black girl's hair changes from a soft silky texture to very kinky before she is about two years old. For mothers of a different race this could be a bit scary and very difficult to adjust to. This metamorphosis that mostly happens with little black girls begins a lifetime of battles with hair that is very difficult to maintain. There will be many years of excruciating scalp pain from daily combing of the hair for the first ten to twelve years. You can make this a lot better for her if you would take a little more time when working with her hair. Slow the process way down.

Little Black Girls Wearing FALSE Hair—Horrific!

I have continued to perform independent research, formulation, and development of hair care techniques with special concentration on problem-solving methods. It disturbs me greatly to see a beautiful black woman with hair that is less than perfect, and it melts my heart to see thousands upon thousands of little black girls whose hair has been totally destroyed. It is my mission and my passion to provide real solutions to the very real hair care issues of mothers and their daughters.

The Question Every Mother Wants Answered

"Is it possible to chemically relax every six, seven, or eight weeks, without scalp burns, without damage, without drying out the hair severely and still get the hair to grow and stay healthy?" YES! But until now this question remained unanswered.

Ironically, GROWING the hair is not the problem, *keeping* the hair on the head after it GROWS is the *real* challenge. It is very much the same for your daughter as it is for you. Every six to eight weeks when it's time for her relaxer retouch there is "new GROWTH." The hair that needs to be relaxed at that point is newly GROWN hair. So as with your own hair, HER HAIR IS GROWING just fine! The recurring problems that you and your daughters are experiencing are hair loss, burdensome dryness, and severe damage. It is the sincere desire of my heart to correct these and many other hair problems.

Take a look around wherever you see black females. Either they are sporting very short boyish haircuts, weaves, wigs, or extensions in the form of braids. Some women have opted for "natural" styles, locs, and the like. I am not condemning these styles. These alternatives are a matter of personal choice, but many of these alternatives cause even more damage. However, the vast majority of women who resort to false hair today do so as a matter of necessity and not as a matter of choice. They believe they have no other choice, but there are many.

I believe you want your own real hair, and I know your little girl does. I say this because I receive e-mails from women all across America, as well as other countries of the world, who voice these sentiments. I know you may find it hard to believe that you can GROW your hair to shoulder length and longer, but it is really possible. I have discovered how to solve the devastating dilemma of severe damage and hair loss. Don't stop reading until you know as much about your hair as this book can teach you.

Is It Really Such a Mystery?

As children you learn to do many things one step at a time. You learn to tie your shoes, brush your teeth, drink out of a glass, and how to dress yourself. Later you learn to tell time, and you learn how to read. Later still you learn how to cook, how to apply makeup, and one day you learn a profession. Everything you've learned started at the beginning and took practice. Then one day you finally knew how to do that particular thing very well.

Learning to handle your daughter's hair has to be done one step at a time. You can learn to care for and handle her hair and yours in the same process. Hair care for black females is a mystery only because until now no one has cared enough to inform you. Your daughter's hair should always be soft to the touch and smell good. It should be healthy, strong, and constantly GROWING. It should have been this way all along. It's the way you want her hair to be. A little girl, a teen, and even a college girl's self-esteem are hampered greatly by having to live each day of their lives with hair problems.

So what are the answers? Products need to be developed that really address specific hair issues. Until then, use the ones endorsed in this book because they WORK! The poor quality products you've been using to care her hair have failed. They simply have not done the job. How do you change it? In all you're getting simply get an understanding.

It is a critical issue of monumental proportion but you now hold the solutions in the palm of your hand. This book is a mother's dream come true. I have discovered solutions that really work. **ShamBOOsie's Hair Wellness Approach to Hair Growth and Hair Care** was formulated to fulfill a mother's total hair care needs by making it possible for your daughter to finally GROW beautiful healthy hair with ease.

Simply put, it WORKS! The key here is compatibility. The design of the product must be comparable to the needs of the hair. My selection of hair products in this book meets this requirement head on. The products must pose a balance between the use of chemical relaxer, the way your hair responds to it, and the way your hair really works.

The products must also meet the hair where it is at the moment, in its present condition and be able to correct as much damage as possible and stop breakage. The products must be able to reverse the extreme dryness and help you keep as much of the hair you and your daughter have, at the same time enabling the both of you to GROW out of the damaged hair into a foot and a half of beautiful healthy new hair in twenty-four to thirty-six months. My selection of products meets these requirements. But none of the products are any good until you learn how to use them properly.

Let the Healing Begin! There is a state-of-the-art concept called **ShamBOOsie's Hair Wellness Approach to Hair Growth**. If you will allow me, I will teach you EXACTLY what each product in this book does for her hair. The system teaches EXACTLY how each product works and what portions to use, because you need to know what to expect. It teaches EXACTLY how to apply every product for the best results, including the chemical relaxer. The objective is GROWTH and healthy hair!

Beautiful Black Hair

Mommies and Baby Care Products

If you are a new mother or mother to be, you probably have discovered the scores of **Baby Care Products** that are available. I would think that you have spent about nine months looking at everything in the stores for babies. In most stores where you shop for the kids are shelves full of baby care products. The problem arises after "the baby years."

You may think that only the hair of **Beautiful Black Baby Girls** changes so drastically and seemingly overnight, but there are females in every race with the same problems of overly curly hair. Managing it is difficult for all of them. It is a mystery to me that such pretty, silky, soft hair is so short lived, and the knotty hair is the only kind of hair in her life that she can be sure of. The real truth is that this problem of tight kinky curls will not change in her lifetime.

She simply will never grow out of it; you haven't. This is the reason she will forever have the arduous task of keeping her hair straight, especially the NEW GROWTH, every six to eight weeks. This is only the beginning of the challenges she will encounter in caring for her hair and keeping it beautiful. My job with this book is to make her job and yours a little easier.

There is no such thing as "children's hair care products." Hair products are made for HAIR! When it comes to shampooing, it is most important to use a shampoo that is also a good moisturizer. All of Nexxus shampoos will meet this requirement. The Humectress Crème Moisturizing Conditioner and Crème Press hairdressing will more than compensate for the other moisture her hair will need. Moisture is the key to settling things down completely with her hair.

Never Experiment with Your Daughter's Hair

The correct selection of hair care products and tools is very important. If you are not sure how to do a chemical application properly or how to use a particular product, leave it alone. One mishap could destroy your daughter's hair, and it could take many years to GROW the hair back. This is why I have made the selections of hair products for you.

Things to Remember

- Do not chemically relax her hair until she can take care of it herself, which will be when she is about ten years old. Never allow your daughter to purchase a home relaxer kit and chemically relax her own hair.
- If you have been using a No-Lye Relaxer STOP. Be sure to follow **The 24 Twenty-Four-Month Hair GROWTH Timetable,** and condition the hair very well before switching to the Lye Relaxer. Apply the chemical to the new GROWTH only, with every retouch.
- Don't allow her to use permanent hair color before age fifteen.
- Heavy oils and grease are no good; use Crème Press Hairdressing instead.
- Never use styling sprays without Crème Press.
- When seeking advice about your child's hair, think what you would do if it was your hair.
- Steer clear from cheap, low quality hair products; they will never work. If you need to save money, don't do so with your hair. Buy the products you need; it's the only way to go.
- Use Crème Press Hairdressing every day no matter what!
- Continue to use baby products until it's time to make the change (about twenty-four months).
- Dudley's Crème Press should always be used to soften her hair while it is still wet or after you dry it. Use as much as you need but only in dime-sized portions.

- Crème Press Hairdressing was originally designed to do hot press and curls, so you can still use it for that purpose. The finished look will be silky and soft. It will be hard to tell the hair wasn't chemically relaxed. When you press the hair using a flat iron and Crème Press, her hair will be much easier to manage for about a week to ten days depending on how well it was done. Practice and learn to do it well.
- **Working with Your Daughters' Hair**
- After the hair has been shampooed and conditioned, spray on some setting lotion and allow it to sit on the hair for about five minutes.
- Towel dry the hair until it's damp. Always begin the drying process when the hair is damp, never dry. If the hair dries before you have the chance to use the blow dryer and comb attachment, have a spray bottle on hand. The spray nozzle on the bottle should spray a light mist, enough moisture to dampen the hair.
- Start by separating the hair into many small sections. You can begin detangling the hair while separating it into the small sections.
- Again, I remind you to begin combing at the ends, holding the hair firmly with one hand between the thumb and fingers to ease the pull on the hair. Comb from the ends of the hair toward the scalp, removing the tangles as you go along.
- Begin the drying process using your blow dryer with the comb attachment, and dry each subsection of hair completely. Make sure the hair is damp to the touch and dry the hair from damp to dry. Plait or braid the hair.
- Move to the next section and repeat the procedure until all of the hair is done. Then plait, braid, or hot press each section of the hair.
- Don't use heavy oils on her hair; the Crème Press will do very well.
- These techniques can be used until the child is seventeen years old or as long as the hair remains natural. The only difference

when the hair is chemically relaxed is the detangling process. The hair will be easier to manage when it is chemically relaxed. It will be safe to chemically relax her hair anytime you decide as long as you care for the hair.

- Use ONLY the conditioners and shampoos mentioned in this book or throw the book away and "do your own thing."

Let's Talk It Over

The idea of kiddie chemical relaxers is just a marketing concept. Some little black girls have hair stronger than yours, and a mild relaxer will have very little effect on the process of straightening their hair. Use a regular relaxer. They are safe, as long as they are not **No-Lye Relaxers**. **Please don't put No-Lye Relaxer in your child's hair.** Remember that a **Conditioning Lye Relaxer** does not come in a kit. You will have to buy the chemical and neutralizing shampoo in separate containers. Select regular strength and use as directed.

Rubber bands and pretty little hair ornaments are safe to use as long as they are not wrapped too tightly. Otherwise the will break some hair and this is something you must avoid doing. Use rubber bands that are one-quarter inch wide and that leave enough stretching ability, so they can be removed easily. Dudley Styling Gel is safe to use in your daughter's hair. Styling gel should leave the hair soft not hard. It should not be used like glue. Dudley Styling Gel will never become flaky. Hair extensions and weaves for little girls are shameful. You must never allow her hair or yours to become so damaged that you have to resort to weaving the hair and hair extensions. They will take out all of her hair and leave bald spots all over her head.

I do understand that you feel you have to do *something* to have hair. But weaves never look that great and everyone knows it's a weave. Most of the ones I have seen are poorly put in. Some are ridiculous and very unattractive. This book will help you GROW your real hair and care for it. You may find it hard to believe that GROWING your hair and hers can be as simple as using the right conditioners and learning to use the chemical relaxer properly. IT REALLY IS THAT SIMPLE! It seems to me that it would be easier to GROW her natural, real hair, and yours too, and the cost to both of you would be much less.

A Great Big Hug from ShamBOOsie

Now give your daughter a Great Big Hug from ShamBOOsie. Do it every time you comb her hair and tell her, "Come and let me give you a great big hug from ShamBOOsie." Do it for me because I love her and her hair very much.

Chemicals and Little Girls' Hair

Today mothers are resorting to Chemical Relaxers very early in hopes of alleviating a rather painful daily hair ritual of having to comb their little girls' hair because it is a dreadful experience for their daughters. But the Chemicals are not getting the job done. There are chemical burns to the scalp, their little girl's hair becomes extremely dry, it pops and breaks constantly, and there are many other Hair Care issues. During the first eighteen years of her life, she will GROW and lose all of her hair dozens of times, but it will only happen because of mistakes her mom will make along the way. The worst mistake is purchasing what I call a **Trick in a Box** (no-lye relaxer) because the makers of this Chemical imply that the product is safe to use. Instead it is the most destructive Chemical on the market. This Chemical will destroy your child's hair. The idea is to learn how to care for her hair, and please know that it's very much the same as caring for your own hair. Just about everything is the same. It doesn't matter that she's a little girl or two years old; Hair Care Products are not age specific.

It disturbs me greatly to see a Beautiful black woman with hair that is less than perfect, and it melts my heart to see thousands upon thousands of little Black girls whose hair has been totally destroyed. It is my mission and my passion to provide real solutions to the very real hair care issues of mothers and their daughters.

- Obstructed Hair Growth—**SOLVED!**
- Extreme Dryness—**SOLVED!**
- Shedding and rapid hair breakage of epidemic proportions—**SOLVED!**
- Scalp Burns from the Misapplication of Chemical Lye Relaxers–**SOLVED!**
- Misapplication of (No-Lye) Calcium Hydroxide Relaxer Kits—**SOLVED!**
- Lack of Hair Care Product Knowledge–**SOLVED!**
- The Use of Substandard Conditioners, Shampoos, and Hair Care other products—**SOLVED!**
- Extremely Undernourished, Unhealthy Hair–**SOLVED!**
- Acquiring Real Hair Growth–**SOLVED!**

I have been able to pinpoint your major areas of concern for your hair and your daughter's hair. You may already be shampooing, conditioning, and chemically relaxing her hair and yours, but you're not doing it correctly. In fact, your efforts are actually destructive. There is an EXACT WAY to handle every aspect of caring for your family's hair. The problem areas have been isolated. All that is needed is to gather the necessary Hair Care products and tools you'll need, and *follow the plan precisely.*

Your daughter needs you to learn the cause of your family's hair problems and how to fix them. I will teach you how to identify the products that are damaging to the hair. This book has listed the products you will need to do the job correctly.

Beautiful Black Hair

My Wildest Dream

My wildest dream is connected to the dreams of millions of black women and their daughters: that they have their own beautiful, long, healthy hair. It is my way to touch and change the lives of millions of black women and their daughters everywhere. I really can make this happen, I can make a difference! I have made many discoveries that will change the way you manage your family's hair.

ShamBOOsie's RELAX and Go-U-Style

Many years ago a friend of mine named Alice owned five Beauty Salons and three Beauty Supply Stores. Alice came up with the idea of offering the public and opportunity to come to one of her five Salons and have their hair Chemically Relaxed for a set price of $24.95. During this time I was offering the service for $95.00, and you could get the service done in many Salons for between $45.00 and $60.00. So the chance to have your hair Chemically Relaxed for $24.95 was a good deal. All of the other Salons Owners in the small town were a bit upset because they were being undercut.

ShamBOOsie's RELAX and Go-U-Style: Gave women of color the chance to have the hair Chemically Relaxed with a **Conditioning LYE Relaxer** for $24.95 but this was the end of the deal. It did not include a Conditioning Treatment, having the hair Wet-Set, Blown Dry and Hot Curled or Styled. It was just the application of the "Chemical LYE Relaxer." The Client would have to return home and STYLE her own Conditioner, Rinse, Wet-Set, Blow Dry and Hot Curl or Style. The Customer left the Salon with her hair wet and under a plastic cap and she was very happy for the savings. If this sounds like a great idea to do in your kitchen or bathroom, Mastering the Art of Application of the Chemical LYE Relaxer is required!

ShamBOOsie's RELAX & Go-U-Style: See the chapter titled A Healthier, Safer, More Comfortable Way to Relax Hair

Ways to Manage the Cost

- Mothers, if you are intending to do the work yourself, Mastering the Art of Application of the Chemical LYE Relaxer is a must. Then shampoo and condition her hair at least ONCE every week. Using ONLY a Chemical LYE Relaxer and use High End Conditioners. Follow this book completely.
- ShamBOOsie's RELAX & Go-U-Style – means that you could do the neighbors' hair, to teach yourself the ART. Once you have Mastered the Art of Application of the Chemical LYE Relaxer, you can teach everyone else in the home who is old enough to learn the application process.
- Schedule the application for each female in the family on a different day.
- Buy your High End Conditioners and Shampoo in larger sizes. Then teach the girls in the family how to use the products properly. Remember, you don't save money by using cheap conditioners—you lose a lot of your hair.
- Don't allow your children under twelve to apply this very dangerous chemical, EVER!
- After you finish RELAXING your daughters' hair, add to the list of things to do…A Great Big Hug from ShamBOOsie…

There are those that believe ShamBOOsie gets a portion of the profits for recommending NEXUS and DUDLEY'S PRODUCTS; you will notice that I am only recommending 2 or 3 products, though both companies make great products! I ONLY recommend what works for ShamBOOsie in the salon.

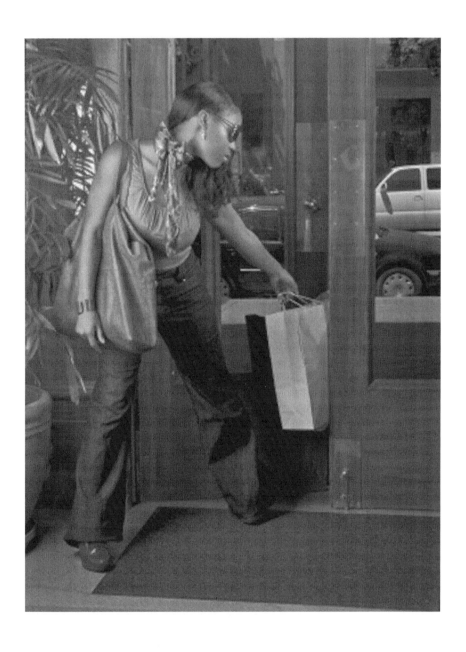

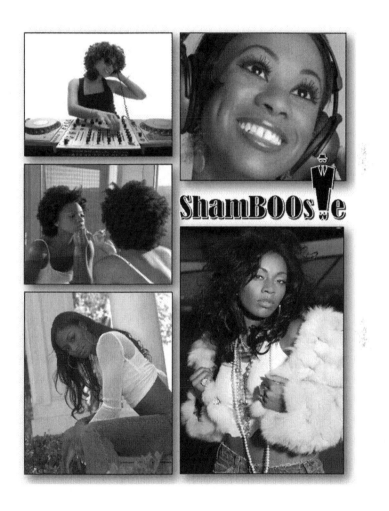

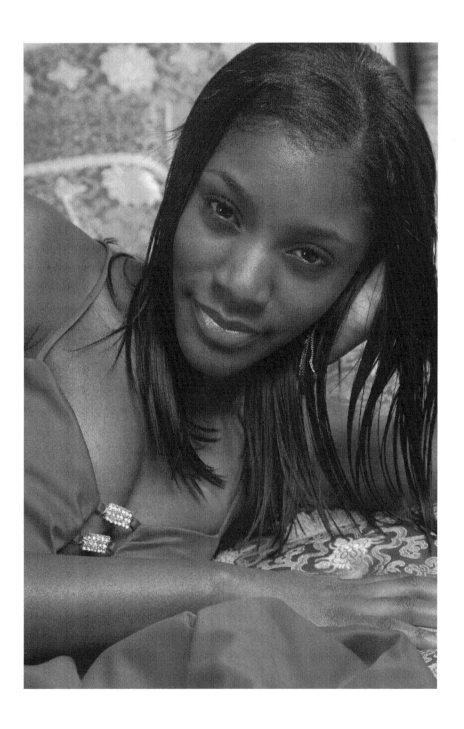

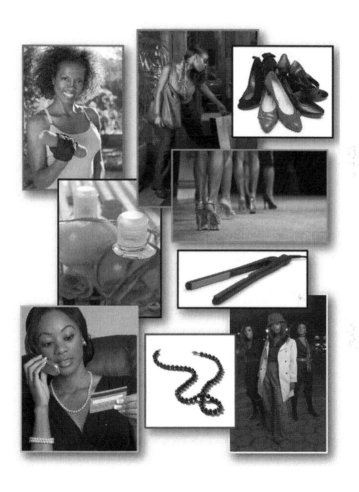

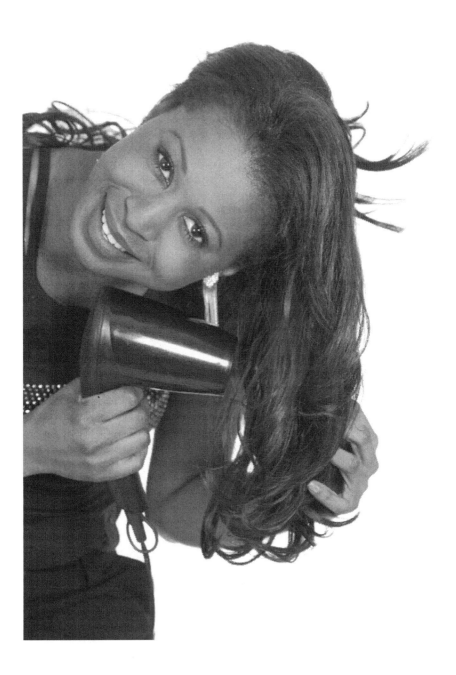

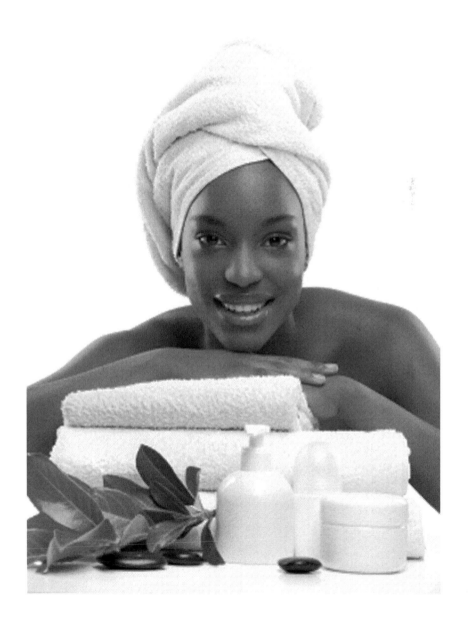

Beautiful Black Hair

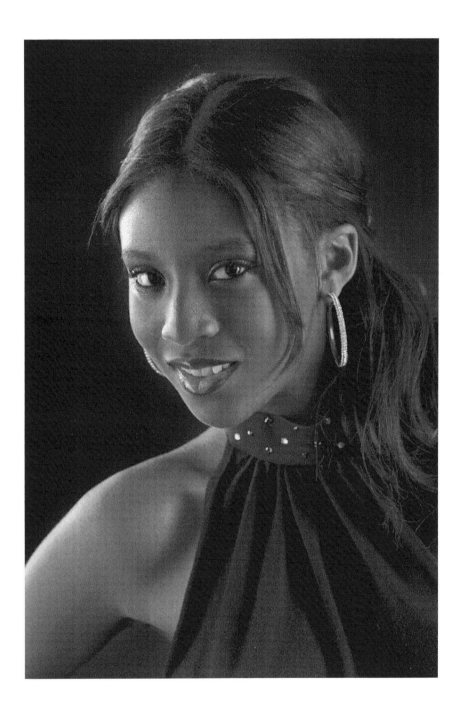

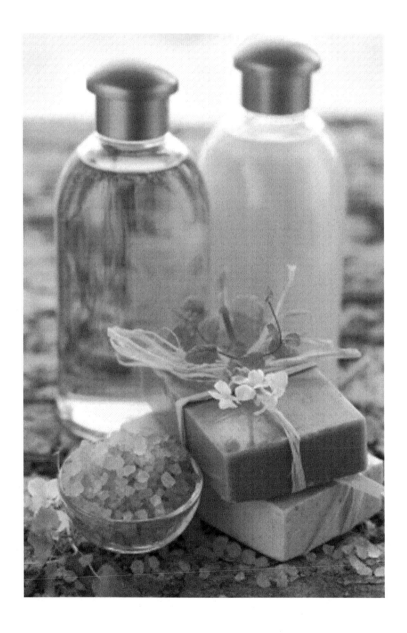

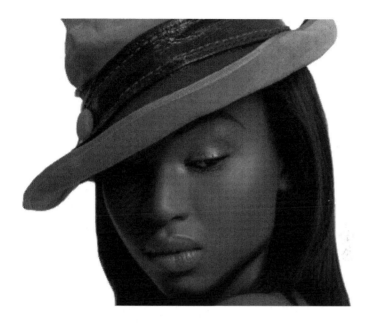

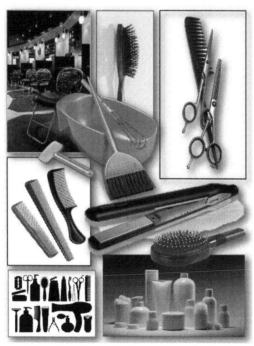

Chapter 8

Conditioners and Treatments

Hair Growth Is All About High-End CONDITIONERS ShamBOOsie's Hair Wellness Approach to Hair Growth The Intensive Hair Care Emergency Section

You Must Perfect the Use of Conditioners

The proper use of conditioners is the secret to getting it right every time! To perfect their use will cause your hair to become very healthy and remain so. I use the phrase **Master the Art** often because anything you do well and have perfected will give you the best results. Part of doing it well is having full knowledge of Conditioners and how they work; with time and study, you'll come to understand their quality and what each type is used for.

Use ONLY White Hair Care Conditioners and Shampoos

There are two most important phases of proper Hair Care that will ensure your hair will GROW longer and healthier than ever. These are the solutions to a "Generational Mystery" of the lack of Hair Growth among black females that has been ongoing for over 2,000 years. The number one most important phase of proper Hair Care is to Master the Application Process of the Chemical Hair Relaxer, which says that your hair must be relaxed only once in the life of the hair. It is possible by applying the Chemical LYE Relaxer to the Newly Grown hair ONLY! You will also need a complete knowledge of the Chemical LYE Relaxer and the Chemical you use for the purpose must be LYE. You can never Self-Apply the relaxer or comb the chemical through the hair.

As I've mentioned, every black woman wonders **How do I chemically relax my hair every six, seven, or eight weeks for the rest of my life and keep my hair healthy, strong, soft, beautiful, and on my head?** Until now, this question remained unanswered. If you are desperately searching for a way to get your hair to grow, **Shamboosie's Hair Wellness Approach to Growing Longer, Healthier Hair** will end that search once and for all. It's the ONLY thing that will work!

Because of the popularity and the use of the **Chemical No-Lye Relaxer Kits,** eight out of ten black females and their daughters from age three to eighty-three are using this most destructive Chemical Relaxer ever created for use on human hair. Your choice of a Conditioner, Shampoo, and Hairdressing is simple—**Humectress Moisturizing Conditioner and Therappe Shampoo** from **Nexxus Products** and **Crème Press Hairdressing** from **Dudley's Products.**

Humectress Moisturizing Conditioner is meticulously formulated with raw materials not found in any other **Moisturizing Conditioner.** When coupled with **Crème Press Hairdressing,** which is applied lightly every day, it alleviates the dryness that comes from combing a No-LYE Relaxer through the hair. Calcium Hydroxide, the chemical in No-LYE Relaxer, damages the hair by causing the dryness. The hair will pop and break until it's all gone. But the **Humectress Moisturizing Conditioner and Therappe Shampoo** (from **Nexxus Products),** and the use of **Crème Press Hairdressing** (from **Dudley's**

Products) are the only things that will alter this extreme DRYNESS. The reason there are only three products on your list of possible Hair Care Products is because they are the only conditioning products in the entire Beauty Industry that are capable of reversing the extreme DRYNESS caused by the **No-Lye Relaxer Kits!** Don't take my word for it—test me and take a good look at your hair. Use these three conditioning Hair Care Products or lose all of your hair, over and over again, year after year.

The Conditioning LYE Relaxer

Where there is only a **Conditioning LYE Relaxer** in your hair, you can use any High-End Hair Care Products on the market such as Nexxus, Redken, L'Oreal, Paul Mitchell Systems, Clairol, or any of the other so-called white hair care products.

Food for Thought

If the manufacturers who make High-End Conditioners and Shampoos were to take their full lines of quality Hair Care Product and put them in Bronze Color bottles and jars, with the face of a pretty black woman on the label, black women would flock to buy them. They wouldn't ask a single question or be concerned about the products being for white hair or black hair. So, go to all the stores where they sell white hair care products and buy $55.00 worth of these quality Hair Care Products. I Prefer Nexxus Products! In plain words: STOP buying using cheap, poor quality or **black hair care products**, they are Hair-destroying products, and they will NEVER, EVER Work!

Learn what you need to know about your hair and Conditioners, Shampoo, Hairdressing, and repeat the same process of application over and over again year round. For this reason you need to "Master the Use of Conditioners" and the use of your all other needed products.

- The Conditioning Shampoos that will clean the hair of all impurities.
- Concentrated Moisturizing Conditioners are for Softness.
- Regular, High-End Protein Conditioners are for Strengthening the hair.
- Concentrated, High-End Protein Conditioners offer additional Strengthening power and should be handled by a Professional ONLY.
- Leave-In Conditioners normally mixed with the conditioning Setting Lotion are for softening the Cuticle Layer of the hair for easier combing when the hair is wet!

Regular use of High-End Quality Conditioners gives your hair the Strength, Softness, Fluffiness, Body, and Bounce of beautiful hair. Your hair should NEVER lie flat against your scalp; it should have body and movement. The magic occurs with the finishing light sheen, Liquids, Gels, Crème Press Hairdressing, and medium hold Styling Sprays. If you use only the best product in every category, you will condition your hair with every application. There is a treatment with every application, which is why they are the true secrets to your success. The cost up front may be more than you are used to, but it will save you hundreds of dollars and ensure real GROWTH down the road.

Quality Conditioners are the keys to REAL GROWTH! The conditioner has to be *superior in quality* and made so that it will work well with **chemically relaxed hair.** There isn't one among the cheaper, poor quality products known as "black hair products!" This does not mean that such superior quality products should only be used on chemically relaxed hair. Conditioners with such a makeup will be great for every other type of hair also. Their uniqueness and higher quality will make them perfect for use on all textures of hair. A selection of just the right conditioners will stop hair breakage, reverse extreme dryness, and give you control of your hair no matter how DRY the hair is.

The right Conditioners will keep the outer layer (the cuticle) resilient and healthy, thereby protecting and strengthening the hair while keeping your hair amazingly SOFT to the touch. Quality Hairdressing, Conditioners, and Shampoo are the only Hair Care Products designed to CARE FOR YOUR HAIR, build body, strength, and softness while keeping your hair in place and GROWING longer.

I Have Taken the Guesswork Out!

With **ShamBOOsie's Hair Wellness Approach to Hair Growth,** all the decisions about Hair Care Products have been made for you; just purchase the items mentioned in this book and use them as instructed. Selecting the right Hair Care Products, especially the Conditioners, can be very difficult, and you have been making many of the wrong choices for some time now. You must understand how each product works to be able to play to win. These products were designed to address each problem you have with your hair. Plus using the right products regularly will prevent most of your Hair Care concerns before they start.

The Price for Quality Is Higher

Growing Strong Beautiful hair is all about **Great CONDITIONERS.** Superior **Hair Care Products** really do work like magic! They will also cost more per unit, but you will spend a lot less over time because they will take better care of your hair. You do not save money by using cheap products. Take a look in your cabinet and see for yourself. Those cheap products don't WORK! If your hair is dry, damaged, breaking, and weak, what you are looking at is the cause not the cure! If I can get you to really understand this, it will make a difference forever in the way you care for your hair.

165

You cannot trade any Conditioner in this PROGRAM for some other, cheaper product and get the same results. It simply is not possible no matter how hard you try. CHEAP hair products cannot work because they were not designed to work in the first place. The notion that all Hair Care Products are the same is ludicrous. This is true even if the ingredients on the label read exactly the same as for professional products. *ALL HAIR CONDITIONERS* are not formulated the same way, *and THEY ARE NOT CREATED EQUAL.* No two manufacturers will make their hair care products the same way. Many women say the same things about Hairdressers and Beauty Salons, but we are not all the same, and all salons are not the same. There are many excellent Hairdressers and Salons.

Take a serious look at the products you have on hand. Pick up each one, and then ask yourself, *"Why do I use this product?"* Don't consult the product's label and answer the question with the label claims. You should know with certainty what every product you use will do for your hair and the results of using that particular product should tell you that it has worked. Let's consider the $9 billion worth of substandard hair products that women of color collectively buy every year. These products haven't done anything to keep your hair healthy, because at the end of every year eight out of ten of you have NO hair. So STOP buying them and STOP using them!

In order to protect your hair and keep it healthy, soft, strong, and beautiful and keep it on your head, you MUST choose a *Conditioning System and always have it on hand.* It is absolutely essential that you learn as much as possible about Conditioners. There is no room for your own opinion or that of anyone else when dealing with your own hair. It is not enough to just use a *good* Shampoo and a *good* Conditioner. Instead it must be a *superior conditioning system* that includes an excellent shampoo designed to do an *EXACT* job. The *conditioning system* you chose must work every time without failure. It must complete the job for which it was created.

A ShamBOOsie Tip:

Conditioners and shampoos are not designed to undo damage or make damaged hair healthy again; nothing can do that. Once the hair is damaged, it must be replaced with new hair. Conditioners and shampoos are not designed to GROW Hair either! Mother Nature grows your hair, and you condition it so that it will remain in place. The Conditioner's job is to *soften* the hair, and it must do *EXACTLY* that. The determining factor is whether or not the hair becomes soft to the touch by the end of the conditioning process. If the hair is breaking, then using a Conditioner that is designed to stop hair breakage must stop the breakage in its tracks.

Let's Talk About Shampoo

There are possibly five different shampoos you could be using at one time or another. They are Regular shampoo, Dandruff shampoo, Neutralizing Shampoo, Clarifying shampoo, and a Prescribed Treatment shampoo. The thing to remember is each shampoo is capable of doing all the work it was designed for in addition to thoroughly cleaning the hair without the aid of the other shampoos.

Clarifying Shampoo

Occasionally when there is a buildup of oil and dirt in the hair, a shampoo with more detergent is needed to strip the hair of everything. A clarifying shampoo is designed to cleanse the hair thoroughly. A clarifying shampoo should be used to address special problems such as buildup of residuals from medication, chlorine, hard water, saltwater damage, oil, grease, and other impurities that can be harmful to the hair and scalp. The idea is to perform preventive maintenance with every application of every product you use. This is why quality is so vital! The clarifying shampoo is NOT designed to treat dandruff.

Regular Shampoo

The regular shampoo is just that, the one you will use before every conditioner. A shampoo should take place every five days to ensure exquisitely clean hair, and it should always be followed with an exquisitely designed conditioner.

Dandruff Shampoo

This shampoo is different from all others. **Dandruff Shampoo** can be used every day, if needed, and the use of this product should be continued until the dandruff has cleared up. **Dandruff Shampoo** contains an ingredient that loosens dry and oily dandruff flakes from the scalp, allowing them to be washed away. If the flakes are dry, choose a shampoo to address that problem, and if oily, the same applies. These shampoos are not designed for anything other than the treatment of dandruff, and should not be used for problems such as eczema, psoriasis, or other skin and scalp conditions. A dermatologist will be able to treat these conditions and should be consulted at the first sign of a problem.

Dandruff Shampoo is a medicated, conditioning shampoo that is mild on the scalp, eliminates dandruff, and stops minor scalp irritation and itching.

Prescribed Shampoo

Keep in mind that a *dermatologist* is a *skin specialist* and is concerned with the scalp, and the *cosmetologist* is a *hair specialist* and is concerned with the hair. If the dermatologist prescribes a special scalp treatment or shampoo, you and your stylist should follow that treatment regimen explicitly until the problem is resolved. Dandruff is often caused by the use of too many chemicals and styling aids or by use of products that are not the right type for your hair and scalp. *Everything* you use on your hair *is a chemical*, in one form or another, including water. Even the wrong kind of water will affect your hair.

Neutralizing Shampoo

Neutralizing shampoos are neutralizer in shampoo form so that they will cling to your hair long enough to neutralize the action of a Chemical Relaxer and STOP it from working. If you don't STOP the Chemical Relaxer from working, it will STOP after it has eaten through every strand of your hair. Neutralizing Shampoo is one of the most important products on your list of things to have on hand. They MUST be understood and used properly, without failure.

The other purpose for the *neutralizing shampoo* is to thoroughly clean the hair. (As you know, the hair is never pre-shampooed the day it is to be chemically relaxed.) The cleaning of the hair must take place during the chemical process. If you were to shampoo, get caught in the rain, go swimming, or wet the hair in any way and then attempt to dry the hair and get a relaxer the same day, your entire scalp would be *"on fire"* in less than five minutes, guaranteed. For this reason, you must always tell your stylist if you have wet your hair within forty-eight hours before getting a relaxer.

Keep in mind that the shampoo, which is part of the formula of this neutralizing product, does not affect the chemical in any way. The shampoo does not *"wash out"* the chemical. It will not stop the chemical from working. Only the *neutralizer* in the shampoo will do that. The *neutralizing shampoo* will not straighten your hair or cause it to revert. It will not dry out your hair or cause breakage, and it does not condition the hair. It will only do what any other shampoo will do, which is clean the hair and clear it of dirt, oils, and other debris.

169

However, its ability to be worked into a thick lather, enables the neutralizer, which is the most important part of the formula, to stay on the hair long enough to terminate the chemical's effect on your hair.

A **Conditioner** is a special chemical agent that is formulated to help restore hair to a natural and healthy state. A conditioner is the key that unlocks the mystery and the secrets to growing beautiful healthy hair. Only when the hair is too far gone is this not possible. Conditioners DO NOT GROW HAIR! They do for hair what a mother does for her babies. Mothers care for, feed, treat every illness (all damage) that rears its nasty head, and protect their babies (the hair).

There are two major types of conditioners—*nonpenetrating* and *penetrating.*

The *nonpenetrating* **conditioner** coats the cuticle layer of the hair with a microfilm coating. These are the most important of all the conditioners because they build strength. The *penetrating* **conditioner** seeps deep into the cortex layer of the hair shaft to restore vital proteins and other minerals. Both types can be used at the same time, and in many cases, they should be.

Conditioners containing concentrated levels of protein should always be rinsed very well, for five full minutes, especially around the hairline and the face (set a timer). These are very dangerous conditioners in the wrong hands. The hair around the hairline and face is usually very dry from daily use of facial soaps that are not designed for use on hair. In most cases, the texture around the face and hairline is weaker, thinner, or smaller in diameter than the hair in the crown and the back of the head. Since this hair is already fragile, the breakage will begin in this area.

You can avoid the breakage by not allowing anyone to do anything to the hair in this area to place extreme tension on this hair, such as braiding or weaving the hair too tightly. This area can easily become bald from pulling the hair too tightly around the face. Mothers do this with their little girls all the time. STOP IT! A **Moisturizing Conditioner** and a daily application of **Crème Press Hairdressing** will help.

The best conditioners contain concentrated levels of protein or moisture. High levels of Protein Conditioners and Moderate Levels of Protein Conditioners are Hair Rebuilders. High quality conditioners, when used regularly, will reduce cuticle roughness and help the hair become stronger, easier to comb, and create a natural shine and softer feel. The microfilm coating that the conditioner leaves on the hair will counteract static electricity so that the hair becomes more manageable. In fact the hair will do everything you need your hair to do much better when it is healthy.

There are many different types of conditioners on the market, and most are designed for a specific purpose. Not all are quality conditioners, and those that are not should be avoided. **(That's about 96 percent of the ones designed to sell to black women).** The secret to successfully treating your hair is in choosing just the right conditioner for the specific hair problem you are experiencing, or if there are no problems, selecting the right ones for regular use. Always use the best that money can buy.

Concentrated Protein Conditioner

(Extremely Dry Brittle Hair Excluded, this will require Concentrated Moisturizing Conditioner with Healing Hydrating Conditioner). The *Concentrated Protein Conditioner* is designed to build strength by hardening the cuticle layer. This is the reason you do not want to put

Beautiful Black Hair

this product of hair that was treated with a No-LYE Relaxer Kit! **The result—Extreme HAIR LOSS!** If you rinse this conditioner well but do not add an additional moisturizing conditioner, drying and styling the hair will create a "straw-like" texture, and the hair will simply break and fall out.

Keep in mind, when choosing conditioners they should also be the right one for your particular hair condition and hair type. For example, if you are conditioning very porous hair (color- treated hair that has a curl or relaxer in it or hair that is extremely damaged) a superior quality protein conditioner should always be used to help rebuild and strengthen the hair.

This is not the conditioner that contains concentrated levels of protein, but normal levels of protein. Heavy crème moisturizing conditioners should be avoided for this type of hair because they will only cause hair in this condition to become even softer and heavier. They will leave the hair limp and getting the final set to hold curls will be very difficult. Instead of a moisture treatment, choose a quality protein conditioner. Concentrated Protein Reconstructor conditioners are deep penetrating conditioners designed to strengthen the hair. It is very important to use these conditioners with caution. In fact, only a professional in a salon should apply these conditioners. If they are not rinsed properly, they will cause more dryness and could do a lot of damage. Always follow up with a Concentrated Moisturizing Conditioner, and only use this kind of conditioning treatment when necessary for an exact reason.

A Treatment Scenario

You go to the salon for a *treatment* because you are experiencing breakage from extreme dryness. Most stylists will reach for a concentrated protein conditioner, which is designed to stop breakage.

172

However, when extreme dryness is the problem, a concentrated protein conditioner *is not* the correct method of treatment because it will harden, strengthen, and rebuild the cuticle layer of the hair. Think about what is happening if your hair is already dry, brittle, and breaking. A concentrated protein conditioner would only add to the problem and cause even more damage and breakage.

This means that if these conditioners are applied to hair that is already dry and brittle, the dryness doubles and even triples, which will also double the amount of the breakage. Although it is best to have these types of treatments performed in the salon, if you must do this at home, there are a few things to keep in mind. Concentrated conditioners will stop most hair breakage, but they should never be used on hair that is very dry and brittle to stop breakage caused by that dryness. There is such widespread use of the **No-Lye relaxer** and only a good heavy moisturizing conditioner will work. In every other case where dryness is not a problem, a concentrated protein treatment can be applied every time you see more shedding or breaking than normal and after every chemical service, which is about every six to eight weeks. Normal shedding is from 50-100 small pieces to full strands of hair a day.

The most important thing to remember is that concentrated protein conditioners should be rinsed for five full minutes or until the hair feels smooth, soft, and silky to the touch. Set a timer, then while rinsing, pay close attention to the hair around the face. It is normally more dry and fragile than all of the other hair, so add an extra portion of moisturizing conditioner in this area.

A Treatment Scenario

You come to the salon for a "treatment" because you are experiencing breakage from damaged hair when a **No-Lye relaxer** is *not* involved, but there is a **Conditioning Lye relaxer** in the hair. The hair is breaking because it is weak and under-conditioned or there is *permanent hair color* in the hair. If you've been using cheap hair products and losing a lot of hair, a **Concentrated Protein Conditioner** could be perfect for hair in this condition. (When a **No-Lye relaxer** is *not* involved!) If permanent **hair color** is **not** in the hair, follow the protein conditioner with a **moisturizing conditioner**.

Treatments: What's The Big Deal?

First determine why the hair needs a *Treatment*. This will help determine which method is best. Breakage should not always be the reason to *treat* the hair. I feel that the term *Treatment* is ambiguous at best and a bit overrated because conditioners are so wonderful these days. When you purchase and use the right ones, there is a *treatment* with every application of every conditioner and product. Regular use of a quality conditioner and shampoo will handle most problems before they ever start. That's what makes **ShamBOOsie's Hair Wellness Approach to Hair Growth** so special. The recommended products are designed to solve many problems as well as prevent them from ever occurring.

A *Treatment* is not always a *Concentrated Protein Conditioner*. This is dangerous to do to your hair if there is a **Chemical No-Lye Relaxer Kit** in the hair. When the hair is in its best condition a regular quality protein conditioner will treat the hair just fine because of the quality of the products. When it comes to intense levels of protein in the form of a conditioner, one of these products is excellent when used properly, but *extremely dangerous* when used incorrectly or on the wrong hair. Therefore, it is best to stay completely away from such products unless you are a Salon Professional.

Sometimes the hair may need *a moisturizing conditioner to stop the breakage*, especially if the problem causing the breakage is DRYNESS.

At other times it may need a mixture of protein and moisture. The **"Treatment"** your hair may need could be just a very good conditioner, which is safe to use every two or three days if you choose. If you really want to treat your hair, be diligent and treat it to regular shampoos and conditioners every week like clockwork with ***High Quality Hair Care Products.*** If you use the right products, the hair receives a treatment with every application. To feel that you need a *Treatment* compels you to purchase something and use it in your hair, not knowing what that product is supposed to do or if the product will do anything at all to solve your problem.

Guessing Games

Guessing games are the reasons you have the problems of shedding, breakage, and your hair is so damaged. Don't guess when it comes to caring for your hair, which is what MOST WOMEN do all of the time. I know what a problem it is to CARE for black hair! At one time or another you have probably purchased a product and said, "I sure hope this stuff works." But if you are reading this book, chances are your products are not working.

Most likely you are *guessing* when you apply ***permanent hair color*** to your hair, so you never get the color you want. You are *guessing* every time you try to relax your own hair, and you could lose all of your hair in as little time as it takes to complete the service. Some of you are *guessing* with your daughter's hair, or your mother's hair, and you are *guessing* every time you walk into a Beauty Salon to have your hair done. Many times Hairdressers are *guessing* as much as you are. Why do you think their hair isn't healthy?

There are ways to always know exactly what you are doing. There is an *exact* way to apply a chemical relaxer and an *exact* way to know which ones are good and which ones are not. There are exactly the right kinds of Hair Color, Shampoos, Oils, Curls, Hairdressings, Chemical Relaxers, Styling Sprays, Gels, and many *exact* types of Conditioners for your hair. If you are going to guess, you should say this to yourself, "I guess I'll take the time to *study* this book, and learn all I need to know to get it right for a change! I guess it is the best way to ensure that I will have beautiful healthy hair."

Moisturizers and Moisturizing Conditioners

Moisture in the hair means softness not wetness. All the Hair Care Products made for use on black hair contain a degree of moisturizers; that's true of even the cheapest ones. This is essential because black hair is always in need of moisture. **Moisturizers** can be found in Relaxers, the Curl, Setting Lotion, Oils, Creams, Hairdressings, in all types of Hair Coloring products, and in many other hair products. This does not mean that all products or all types of moisturizers are suitable for your hair. And it does not mean that a given product is okay to use just because there is moisture in its formula. It does mean that black hair lacks moisture more than anything else. Your hair needs a unique type of moisture that will keep your hair soft at all times. Heavy oils will not do!

The moisture your hair will need on a daily basis should be subtle, light enough not to weigh the hair down, and **provide moisture that will last all day**. A woman's hair should be **so soft to the touch,** and it should always smell good. Achieving this moisture is what you should be trying to accomplish every time you service your hair, even if you set your hair on rollers.

Leave-In Conditioner

A **leave-in conditioner** speaks for itself and can be used as often as you choose. However, the leave-in conditioner does not take the place of the regular conditioner. The process should be: shampoo, rinse, apply regular conditioner, rinse, apply leave-in conditioner, apply setting lotion, and then style as usual. The leave-in conditioner can be mixed with setting lotion or sprayed in before every comb out and set.

A ShamBOOsie Tip:

Fantastic Body Setting Lotion by **Dudley** will do exactly the same thing, plus it's the best setting lotion there is. This product must be applied after every shampoo and conditioner, before the hair is air dried or blown dry.

Level Ten: A Higher Standard of Excellence

Imagine the health of your hair on a scale from one to ten with Level ten being the healthiest your hair can be. In order to have the healthiest hair at Level ten, all of the hair care products you use must also be at Level ten. Level one or Level three hair care products will never perform at Level ten, no matter how often you use them.

The hair care products you use, the tools you use, and the level of training and skills of the hairdresser should ALL be at Level ten. Likewise, the beauty salon you select must be a Level ten salon. I have to admit finding a competent professional will take some time and research, but they are out there.

If your desire is to care for your hair at home, the process is determined by your sincere desire to do the work. Your knowledge of how to properly care for your hair must also be at Level ten. This will require educating yourself, which is what this book is designed to do. Anything less than Level ten in any of the areas spells failure. So if you are willing to do the work, *ShamBOOsie's Hair Wellness Approach to Hair Growth* will supply you with all the tools. Simply follow the directions and watch the magic happen.

Speaking of quality and protection, about 90 percent of the products made for use on black hair are substandard and incapable of protecting the hair. This is one of the reasons women of color and their daughters are having so many hair problems. As I mentioned earlier, there are only two categories of hair care products—good and bad. Ethnicity has nothing to do with it.

Strength + Softness = GROWTH

Strength plus Softness equals GROWTH, but the hair has to be serviced often for this to work. The perfect *Conditioning System* is the *"glue"* that holds the hair together and keeps it from falling out. Selecting the right Conditioners is essential to GROWING SOFTER, STRONGER, BEAUTIFUL, and HEALTHY hair.

The **Conditioner** is a *strength builder* and no other product is capable of doing the job of the conditioner. Always remember that the hair absolutely has to be fed a minimum of every 3-5 days with a Shampoo and quality Conditioner, and *every 4, 5, or 6 weeks with a **Concentrated Conditioner**. The Conditioner* should be one that will always address the needs of the hair at the moment of application. **ShamBOOsie's Wellness Approach** makes this easy for you.

All you need to do is study this book, learn as much as possible about your hair, and apply what you have learned. It's that simple! I could give you a fish or teach you how to fish, which is much better. I could give you a quick fix or teach you how to really care for your hair, which is your best chance of acquiring or GROWING BEAUTIFUL hair, and maintaining it for the rest of your life.

You Must Remember This: There is absolutely nothing you can ever do to make level two Hair Product performs at level ten. So use ONLY level ten Quality Hair Care products. It should be that way with everything you buy, if possible! The quality and condition of your hair will always be maintained at the exact level of the quality your Hair Care Product is capable of. This is true whether you select the products or your hairdresser selects the products. The majority of products made for use on black hair and most of what is used in the black hair salons falls in the category between level zero to level four at best. These products will actually create more problems for your hair. The cost to you over a period of time can be astronomical both financially and personally.

Picture This!

This is how most people of every race view Hair Care Product. Imagine walking into a Beauty Supply Store. On all of the shelves are containers with no brand names, just bottles, jars, and cans with a single words on bright colored labels. On one shelf bottles are labeled with the word *SHAMPOO*, others are labeled *CONDITIONER, SETTING LOTION, HAIRDRESSING, RELAXER,* and so on. There are no descriptions or instructions for use on the containers. All of them are very cheap and you get a lot for your $3.50. None of them are designed to do your hair any good, and no one has made you aware of it. All of the words on the labels are printed in large, bold, black, capital letters like **HAIR SPRAY!** You purchase what you need, go home, and use it on your hair. No matter how much or how often you use these products, they do *nothing* for your hair.

Now back to reality. If I were to ask how often do you shampoo and condition your hair, using the products you have on hand, you might answer "once a week or once every two weeks," or some such thing. All the while your hair is still dried out, lifeless, and falling out by the handful. You could be making all the right moves of the dance but wearing the wrong shoes or applying shampoo and condition every week but using substandard products.

Beautiful Black Hair

No one to this day has told you that the conditioner is supposed to keep the hair strong, stop the breakage, and help your hair grow soft and BEAUTIFUL. This is what should take place, but only if they really do work, only if you use the **EXACT** ones needed for your hair, and use them often enough. However, once every two weeks will never do the job. Shampooing and conditioning the hair should take place every four to five days with quality hair care products.

Black Hair Care Products

The products you have been using, so-called black hair care products are easily identified by their containers displaying bright labels with single words, written in large black lettering. Therein is the source of all your hair problems. You must change your thinking and choose the products that are best for your hair regardless of their labels.

The Global Beauty Giant L'Oreal Paris

As I mentioned earlier, L'Oreal Paris makes both the Black Hair Care Products and what is perceived to be known as White Hair Care Products! For BEAUTIFUL hair, you need level ten products, regardless of who you think makes the products. When it comes to purchasing your Conditioners and Shampoos, buy and use ONLY those for white hair. I suggest Nexxus. You may be surprised to learn that very few of the so-called black hair care products are manufactured by black people. Most are owned and made by **L'Oreal Paris.** The makers of these products find other ways to bait you and get you to purchase their products. They place the picture of a pretty black woman on the box, name the product after the job it is supposed to do, use wording like "No Lye," and insinuate that products are made for specific ethnicities. Nothing could be further from the truth.

I am not saying that all of the products these companies make are not good enough to truly take the best care of your hair; many of

them are. High-End white hair care products are the best for use on black hair and everyone else's hair! I am saying don't choose your hair care products based on the color of your skin because you will lose your hair. You must purchase product that is ten times as good as what you have been using. Please move beyond purchasing products by brand names, unless those brand names are synonymous with Superior Quality Hair Care Products.

Why Quality Hair Care Products?

Many of you will read this book and say to yourselves, "He keeps saying the same things over and over again. It's use High-End Hair Care Products and STOP using the Chemical No-Lye Relaxer Kits!" These are the two most difficult things to get women to comprehend. A thousand women will have a thousand different opinions about the type of product they use on their hair. They all can't be right. In fact most of them are wrong. The products in this book are a selection from the crème of the crop. They were made to work every time.

This book is not about selling hair care products; it is about making your hair healthy and beautiful. It is about *GROWING* your hair, which is something that most black women believe, is impossible to do. The most wonderful thing about these **Quality Hair Care Products** is they will do above and beyond what you can imagine to keep your hair soft, beautiful, healthy, and *GROWING* strong. The more you use the right products the right way, the better the products will work, and the stronger, healthier, and more beautiful your hair will *GROW.*

You can trust this book and all that it says. You can trust the products listed because each of them is excellent and so much better for your hair. I use the slogan ShamBOOsie: the name you can trust! You can really trust me because I really care about your hair! There is a compilation of about nine different products I have put together to take back and maintain control of the overall health of your hair.

Though you may not use all of these products at the same time, these are the products you should have in your Hair Care First Aid Kit. It is imperative that you have a collection of each of these Conditioners on hand at all times. This way when a need presents itself, you can address the need immediately. Once you have such a full line of superior quality products, the next thing is to master the use of the product line.

In Good Condition

If I can change the way you think about conditioners, I can change everything you are experiencing with your hair. You must stop thinking "Black Hair Care Products," and to start thinking "Quality Hair Care Products." Only the best conditioners will revitalize, energizer, nourish, infuse nutrients, improve manageability, and stimulate the hair shaft. *Conditioners* perform the truest form of therapy for your hair. The way to determine what is best for your hair is simply to **"Allow the hair *to dictate.*"** Extreme Dryness in the Hair = Extreme Hair Loss. **Reverse the Dryness and Stop the Breakage!** Dryness, even a normal degree of dryness, will create an environment for hair breakage.

The solution is to take back control of the extreme dryness, reverse the affect it is having on your hair, and maintain control of all forms of dryness. You must also be aware that there are many other reasons and ways your hair can become weak, damaged, and fall out. I talk so much about dryness because it is the major reason women are losing so much hair. The objective is to choose the right ones to render the hair soft with styling ability. You want the hair soft, but you also want the hair to hold whatever style you choose to wear.

A ShamBOOsie TIP:

Your hair cannot possibly remain healthy if you only shampoo and condition once or twice per month. If the product you are using is of poor quality, the damage will increase tremendously. Many of you tell me you are shampooing and conditioning your hair once a week. If your hair looks, feels, and reacts to the neglect by becoming weak and falling out, it should tell you that what you are using in your hair is not working. The best conditioners are designed to work very well.

In her comments about my previous book, a reader said that I was suggesting the use of *expensive* hair care products. Well, she is right in thinking the products I am recommending will cost you more money. Isn't the thought of having beautiful healthy hair worth every dime you will spend on *quality* hair care products if they really work? Using cheap shampoos and conditioners + applying your own chemicals, (Hair color, Curls, Bleach, and Relaxers) + letting the hair go for days, weeks, and, in some cases, months = badly damaged, weak, broken hair. Need I say more?

Why Is It So Dangerous to Have Dry Hair?

What's for Dinner? You are probably wondering what food has to do with hair care. To better illustrate the danger of dry hair, allow me to use a food illustration right here.

Imagine you are preparing a spaghetti dinner. The uncooked spaghetti in this scenario represents your hair in its driest state. The thing to remember is that ***extreme dryness*** in hair requires the treatment of an ***extreme moisturizer*** to remove or reverse the dryness and render the hair *"baby soft."* Such moisturizing products are not so easy to come by. Most that are on the market do not work. Because the dryness is *"extraordinary,"* the treatment must also be *"extraordinary."*

183

So, the pot of boiling hot water is bubbling away on the stove in anticipation of the pasta. A small amount of oil is added to the mix, to keep the spaghetti from sticking together. The oil mixed with the boiling hot water is the perfect solution for softening and preparing the very dry spaghetti. Then you would take several sticks of dry uncooked spaghetti in both hands, break them in half, and drop them into the oil and boiling hot water. This is quite easy to do because the sticks of spaghetti are very dry and brittle. The uncooked pasta will break with little or no effort. So will your hair in the same condition. In about five minutes, the once very dry, brittle uncooked spaghetti will be so soft you will be able to wrap it around your finger. The spaghetti will now bend easily instead of breaking because of the moisture from the hot water.

Now think about your dry hair for just a moment. A superior quality *moisturizing conditioner* **applied six times in four-day intervals will take control of the dryness and strengthen the hair. The combined efforts of all four conditioning products**—Therappe Moisturizing Shampoo, Humectress Moisturizing Conditioner, and Keraphix Strengthening Conditioner from Nexxus Products, and the Superior Crème Press Hairdressing from Dudley's Products—**properly applied at the scheduled intervals, will reverse and control the dryness caused by the destructive** No-Lye Chemical Relaxer **and other drying chemical processes.**

The **Styling Spray** lets you determine how much hold you need in your hair depending on how full your curls are. The alcohol content of **Styling Spray** is very small. Therefore, when it is used correctly in conjunction with the **Crème Press Conditioning Hairdressing**, it will never dry the hair out. Growing Strong Beautiful hair is all about **Great CONDITIONERS**. High Quality **Hair Care Products** really do work like magic!

Color Changes Everything

Once **permanent hair color** goes into chemically relaxed hair, it becomes a double chemical process, and the methodology of shampooing and conditioning your hair changes dramatically. It is a matter of selecting and applying a superior **Protein Conditioner**. The products within **ShamBOOsie's Hair Wellness Approach** have been designed to handle this change in the texture of your hair. The rest is simply a matter of the closeness in timing of each application of the conditioners, especially before and immediately, after the color application.

The key here is to use a *permanent hair color* that has *no ammonia* in its formula. I recommend that all color applications designed to lift the natural color of your hair be administered by a Salon Professional. With today's technology coloring hair is a precise science.

With a Conditioning LYE Relaxer, I can safely relax a white woman's hair. The belief that No Lye is better than Lye Relaxer has caused women of color to lose a lot of hair, and it has collectively cost them billions of dollars each year. It has also forced them to resort to replacing their real hair with different configurations of Synthetic Hair Fiber (**false hair**).

The Strong Arm of the Conditioner

Hair is 98.9 percent protein, so what kind of conditioner do you want to use most often? You want to use a *protein moisturizing conditioner* whose job is to give the hair back some of its strength. This is accomplished by infusing the hair with the protein it loses over time and especially after being permanently colored, permed, and/or relaxed. The conditioner will also feed the hair and fill it with many of its wonderful natural properties.

Beautiful Black Hair

A ShamBOOsie Tip: Even the best *protein conditioners* may not stop the hair from falling if you do not allow the *neutralizing shampoo* to complete its job of stopping the action of the chemical. See chapter on Proper Chemical Relaxer Application.

Holding Agents

The job of the *setting lotion* is to soften the cuticle layer so the hair will comb easier. It also acts as an artificial bond to help the hair hold its curl in a dry set or when the hair is blown into style with blow dryer and round brush. This set will last two to three days depending on the condition, strength, and texture of the hair. Remember that the natural bonds, which cause your hair to hold curl on its own, were destroyed during the relaxing process. If your hair is to ever hold a curl after it has been relaxed, you will need an artificial bonding product— a holding agent such as *setting gel, hair spray, spritz, mousse, or setting lotion* and a hot curling iron.

Growing Strong Beautiful Healthy Hair is all about **Great Conditioners.**

Superior Hair Care Products really do work like magic!

Chapter 9

Wearing FALSE HAIR Has Its Downfalls

Many black women and their daughters are either wearing FALSE HAIR, have very short hair, or have badly damaged hair. FALSE HAIR, whether tightly braided, glued, bonded to one's hair and scalp, or woven by being sown to small braided sections of hair using false or synthetic hair, is often very difficult to manage. With FALSE HAIR there is no way to keep the real hair shampooed and conditioned or keep the scalp and hair clean. The most important part of managing your hair is CONDITIONING the hair. It is the ONLY way to keep your hair strong and healthy and to stop breakage and keep the hair soft to touch. Some women believe they can go for months without doing anything to their hair and scalp.

Wearing a weave does not stop the hair from Growing. Even with braids and weaves the hair still must be Chemically Relaxed every six, seven, or eight weeks like clockwork. Do you realize that you are relaxing your hair because it is GROWING? In addition, wearing the hair too tightly braided for long periods causes breakage in large patches. Add to this, the use of **No-Lye Relaxer**, combing relaxer through the hair with every application. Then there's the use of substandard Hair Products. All of these are causes of hair damage and hair breakage. In the end as with every year that passes black women collectively spend $9 BILLION on hair products but have no hair to show for it. (Notice that I avoided using the term **Hair CARE Products**.)

The Damage Is Extreme but Correctable with Time

The problems of continuous and rapid hair loss are about the same for women of color and their daughters, as young as four years of age, around the world. There are several reasons for this tragedy. For many it seems there is no help in sight, and it seems that much of the damage cannot be repaired. **The GROWTH is replenishing!** Presently, the only choice for more than 85 percent of these women is to wear some form of False Hair or to live with the idea of having the hair continue to fall out. There is nothing wrong with your real hair, the problem is that you have not learned how your hair works, and you insist on buying the cheap products marketed as **Black Hair Care Products!** STOP right NOW! Start buying and using **white hair care conditioners and shampoo products from Nexxus!** You are allowing someone who doesn't care one bit about your hair to create many complete lines of the poorest products on the planet and sell to you. They do not work and were never formulated to work, in the first place.

Can you imagine a four-year-old little black girl wearing false hair? The sad reality is that this is happening with women of color all over the country and around the world. There are millions of women searching online discussion groups and chat rooms, bookstores, magazines, libraries, and beauty supply stores, hoping to find solutions to their numerous hair care problems. The solutions in this book will put an end to their search and reverse this seemingly infectious Hair Disease.

What has caused most of their hair care problems is the use of SUBSTANDARD HAIR CARE PRODUCTS. Nearly 100 percent of the products they are buying are either substandard or not made to directly address their problems. They simply do not work; products that do WORK are referred to as white hair care products! Remember that your product choices shouldn't be guided by skin color/ethnicity. Products continue to be marketed to different ethnic groups, but don't fall for it. Avoid the trick in a box chemical relaxer called **"No-Lye"** or **"Sensitive-Scalp Relaxer"** because it is responsible the most, nearly 90 percent of black women's problems. Right now at least 90 percent of the 20 million black women in the country are using this cheap product and dealing with some type of hair care dilemma. The greatest problem is keeping the hair strong, healthy, and on the head. Managing black hair is like trying to open a combination lock without the knowledge of the numbers. I want to give you the EXACT combination to unlock this age-old mystery--ONLY Humectress Moisturizing Conditioner, Therappe Shampoo (NEXXUS) and the best Hairdressing EVER Cream Press Pressing Oil (DUDLEY'S) DRYNESS be gone!

If Possible You Must Return to the Salon for Services

Many black women say that the use of Superior Hair Care Products and visiting the salon for service is too expensive. Many of them have asked me if there are cheaper products that will work as well. They already have the answer to that question. The value of your hair should be what is more important, not the cost of Superior Hair Care Products. If you decide to go with cheap hair products, you need to know that you will spend twice as much as the cost of Superior Hair Care Products because your hair will become more damaged, and you will spend much more trying to keep your hair from falling out. Cheap Hair Products will never WORK!

Superior Hair Care Products: The Kit Ain't It!

If you see a dress, a purse, or a pair of shoes and you say to yourself, "I must have that," nothing will stop you from getting the money to buy that dress, purse, or pair of shoes. There is no substitute for quality especially when it comes to buying Superior Hair Care Products for your hair. You can't afford **NOT** to use quality hair care products and you **CAN** afford regular visits to the salon for services. You cannot afford to continue "Self-Applying the Chemical No-Lye Relaxer Kit" at home—**The Kit Ain't It!**

I get requests for recommendations from women everywhere who are desperately searching for knowledgeable Salon Professionals to care for their hair. Your cares and feelings are also involved, and I understand that you are finding it very hard to trust our profession again because we have let you down so many times. It is simply a matter of education and training, especially about the proper application of the chemical relaxer. The system of relaxer application I have used for many years is nearly flawless and more comfortable for the client because there is no burn sensation ever!

ShamBOOsie's Hair Wellness Approach to Hair Growth is a STOP and READ proposition. You must STOP doing everything you have been doing to your hair, including **"Self-Applying Chemical Relaxer."** It breaks my heart to see women of color and their little girls with badly damaged hair. You need to LOOK into the possibility that there is a better way to handle you family's hair without spending a lot of money. Then LISTEN to **ShamBOOsie** and trust him; what do you have to lose? Use **ShamBOOsie's Hair Wellness Approach to Hair Growth**. Don't add or take away any part of it, and it will work for you. You will learn that you can GROW your hair longer and more beautiful than ever. Even if you don't want long hair, I'm sure you want your hair to be healthy. **ShamBOOsie's Hair Wellness Approach to Hair Growth** is NOT just another hair care system; this one was designed to DO the JOB, and it WORKS.

Trust...

When there is a solid bond of trust between the consumer and the stylist, the rest is Success with a capital S and everyone is happy! The key to the success of any salon operation is an ongoing system of education and training in every area of service. This is very much a part of **ShamBOOsie's Hair Wellness Approach to Hair Growth.** It is **ShamBOOsie's** intention to put such a program in place. But the education process begins with you. You must make a commitment to care for your hair, and then your hair will reward you with real GROWTH.

I'm a Hair Watcher!

In the early 1960s there was a popular song called **"I'm a Girl Watcher."** If you were to become a "Hair Watcher" you would notice immediately that eight out of ten black women, young and old, regardless of economic status, are wearing some form of **false hair**. To demonstrate the severity of the problems, nearly every black woman in America has many of the same hair care problems; hardly anyone is exempt. Many well-known celebrities and even millionaires **MUST** wear **false hair** to have hair. This is nothing new for entertainers who travel and perform every night, but under those wigs and hairpieces is damaged, broken hair.

It is very sad but true, no matter how much money the black woman makes, she stills believes there is such a thing as black hair care products, and that belief is an obstacle to the possibility of her ever having healthy hair. There are only "good" and "bad" hair care products. She has allowed someone to put a **No-Lye Relaxer** in her hair, thinking it's better and safer. Her hair still becomes extremely dry and falls out by the handful. Therefore, she has to have someone weave, braid, bond, or attach some form of **FALSE HAIR** to replace it.

The Black Woman's Hair Problems Don't End in the USA!

Women of color in other parts of the world are also victims. Recently, I traveled to Germany, London, and France, where I found that black women and their daughters are wearing **False Hair also.** It's happening all over the world! So what is the common denominator? It is the use of the **No-Lye Relaxer—a Dehydrating Monster!** It is unbelievable that this chemical has traveled around the world, destroying every head of hair in its path.

Some women still believe the myth that wearing **False Hair** will actually make their hair grow. Somehow they don't believe that their hair is **growing all the time!** Wearing weaves, braids, locks and twists are trends that can cost big bucks. The Black Beauty Salon business is still the largest black-owned business in the country. Yet the salons have lost nearly 80 percent of their business because of the **No-Lye Relaxer**, poor quality products, and the use of **False Hair**. Many salon owners have opted to convert their salons to braiding and weaving establishments, just so they can stay in business. **ShamBOOsie's Hair Wellness Approach to Hair Growth** will change this by helping to rebuild the trust!

Never before in the history of the BLACK WOMEN has it been possible to HOT PRESS or CHEMICALLY RELAX the hair, keep it healthy and strong, and most importantly, KEEP THE HAIR ON THE HEAD AND GROWING. Even if there were no chemicals used in the hair it   it would still fall out.

ShamBOOsie's Hair Wellness Approach to Hair Growth is a concept that lets you CHEMICALLY RELAX the hair and keeps it on the head. If there is any doubt, simply put this theory to the test. This is revolutionary, cutting edge technology.

192

The Solution to the Dryness!

ShamBOOsie's Hair Wellness Approach to Hair Growth contains the solution to the problem of EXTREME DRYNESS! Without this System the DRYNESS and the BREAKAGE will persist until all the hair is gone. This is exactly what's happening at this very moment.

When do the hair challenges for the black female begin? As I explained earlier, starting at about eighteen to twenty-four months of age the hair of most black babies goes through a metamorphosis. That change begins a lifetime of emotional hell for these "Little Brown Beauties." The never-ending process of trying to keep the hair straight creates a difficult challenge, and the pain from combing her tightly curled hair is very hard to deal with. She must live with the problem for the rest of her life. (Ask any black woman, and she will agree.)

The problem becomes even more critical when a child has to wear **FALSE HAIR** because the mother has no choice when trying to relieve the pain but to comb a No-Lye Relaxer through the hair. Little Black Girls should not have to wear **FALSE HAIR** to have hair; it makes no sense! It is extremely painful to comb kinky hair. In fact, it hurts so badly that many mothers report that their daughters will start to cry even before the hair combing ritual begins and will continue to cry until it ends. The horror these "Little Brown Beauties" go though, the **FALSE HAIR**, the breakage, and the embarrassment they must contend with was my inspiration for writing books about hair care. As a professional, I knew that something could be done about it, and so I set out to do something about it!

The reason there is such widespread use of the **No-Lye Relaxer** to chemically straighten is because women have experienced first-degree burns to the scalp from the misuse of the **Lye Relaxer,** and they really believe that **No-Lye** is safer. So in an effort to prevent the scalp burns, they turned to the **No-Lye Relaxer**. If the product were to remain in the jar, with the cap on tightly, there would be no way the chemicals could cause dryness, breakage, or burn your scalp. So the problem is not with the chemical itself; the error lies with the person applying the chemical. It is simply a lack of know-how!

Today they call this chemical a "sensitive scalp" relaxer, but there is nothing "sensitive" about this chemical. Either way, **No-Lye Relaxer** is the worst most destructive product ever made for use on black hair! You don't have to buy it for your kids because they are buying it and using it on their own hair with tragic and inexcusable results. It is a shame that this poison's popularity has grown over the past twenty years. Thankfully, this is starting to change.

You want your hair to GROW, but to do so you must also be able to have your hair chemically relaxed and keep the hair healthy and strong through six applications of the chemical each year, for as long as you wear your hair relaxed. This could be twenty to forty years or longer! Only the best and highest quality conditioners and shampoos will make this possible. Nothing else will work! Of course, a proper application formula is also required.

By teaching the many formulas and using the superior hair care products, **ShamBOOsie's Hair Wellness Approach to Hair Growth** can establish a trust that will last for generations to come. My devotion to better hair care is the basis and primary focus of my practice as a Professional Hair Care Practitioner. The SCIENTIFIC RESEARCH that went into **ShamBOOsie's Wellness Approach to Hair Growth** was more than twenty years in the making. I believe that personalized preventive care is of the utmost importance in achieving healthy hair-growth goals. My education and experience in the Cosmetology field has enabled me to incorporate a client-centered approach to hair care that is tailored to the unique needs of the individual. I have also taken into consideration the emotional aspects involved in order to make an accurate diagnosis of their hair care needs.

I believe that knowledge is empowering. When Salon Professionals and black women in general understand hair care and the mechanisms that cause injury, they will become more committed to doing what it takes to fix the problems. It makes good business sense. I am devoted to educating women about ethnic hair care solutions. There are literally hundreds of products that claim to deal with hair loss and growth but few can actually prove their efficacy, or have any study to back up their claims. Hair **growth** was never the problem. **Keeping the hair that is grown** healthy, even while chemically relaxing, is the real challenge. **ShamBOOsie's Hair Wellness Approach to Hair Growth** will help you maintain the health, growth, and beauty of your hair for years to come.

Chapter 10

The Color of Hair: Understanding the Science of Coloring Hair

Hair Coloring as it **relates to black hair or Chemically Relaxed Hair!** *Mother Mary had a little black girl whose hair was white as snow, and every time she colored her hair, her white hair continued to GROW!* But this is a GOOD thing and the perfect way to notice that the hair is GROWING.

I have seen many lovely shades of gray, and it can be quite beautiful on some people, although in reality, most people would like to rid themselves of every white and gray strand. Whether you desire to cover, color, blend, or flaunt your gray hair, I hope the information and advice stated here will help you do it beautifully. Do yourself a favor and **"Learn to LOVE your hair as much as you LOVE yourself."** Only when you truly LOVE your hair will you do all that is needed to grow it beautifully and keep it that way. **Conditioning is the key!**

This is the true story of a lovely sixteen-year-old black girl who had naturally white hair that she had been coloring most of her young life. Like many, she used "jet-black" permanent hair color every three to four weeks. Hair usually turns gray with age, but when it happens to a young person, it can be difficult to deal with, to say the least.

This young girl is probably about twenty-five years old now, and chances are she is still spending a lot of money on hair coloring. The good news is that she, and others like her, can wear their hair any color they choose, and there are many color options. Many entertainers in today's pop culture are wearing a rainbow of colors—a trend that has become commonplace.

Have you ever heard the phrase Men don't like roots? What it means is after having their hair colored, men don't like to see the return of gray hair at the scalp, which is the new growth. Believe me when I tell you that women don't like roots either.

True Story...

I was watching a news article on TV about a black woman who had just given birth to a beautiful baby boy. The reason the news media decided to tell this couple's story was because the father had a white patch of hair in the front of his head. You are probably saying to yourself, so what, that's no big deal. The news people turned the camera on the newborn and low and behold, the baby had the same white patch of hair in the front of his head.

The Quantity of Gray Hair is the Determining Factor

Never relax hair you have just colored or any hair that has color in it. The hair isn't strong enough, which is why you must apply the chemical to the New Growth ONLY! Always Color the hair after it has been Chemically Relaxed. The one thing a black woman must contend with on regular basis is the **Chemical Relaxer Application every six to eight weeks** and it MUST be done on time. Somewhere around age thirty-five she may start to see a few gray strands, which will increase with time. At some point most women consider coloring and relaxing the hair, just remember to RELAX FIRST! I refer to this as *double processing*. The hair will be changed tremendously depending on whether she *covers* the gray or *colors* the gray the same color as her natural color. Or she may choose to change her hair color altogether. Just getting rid of a few gray strands of hair will require the lesser amount of change in the texture of the hair, because covering a few strands can be done with a coater, temporary, or water-base color.

This may require a permanent color applied quickly to all the hair. The chemical will remain on the hair for about ten minutes, after first allowing the mixture of color to remain in the bottle for about ten minutes to oxidize in the bottle with the cover off. Once the color changes in the bottle apply it to all the hair as quickly as possible, wait ten minutes and rinse well, condition the hair without shampooing the hair, style and finish. If she is looking to completely change the color of her hair, this will require the greatest change in the texture of the hair and MUST be done by a professional colorist. Seek a **white hair stylist and colorist** because they have more experience coloring hair—unless it's ShamBOOsie. Be sure to seek an *experienced* colorist.

Gray hair in and of itself is much stronger and more resistant than the normal hair that has color. Coloring the gray when it is more than 30 percent of the hair you have means that you will have to color all of the hair in order to get rid of the Gray or White hair. The fact that Gray hair is resistant could be in your favor if you have no intentions of covering or coloring the hair. If you choose wear/ flaunt your Gray or White hair, you have a much better chance of GROWING a longer, stronger, healthier, softer, lovelier head of hair. This also means there will only be one chemical in the hair (the Relaxer), as opposed to having two chemicals, Permanent Hair Color and Relaxer, which we call *double processing*.

This is How ShamBOOsie Does It:

- Every chemical service must be on an exact schedule, especially Coloring the Hair
- The chemical employed must be exactly the right kind of coloring product for your hair and it MUST work very well with the Chemical Relaxer, meaning that you don't want the color to change the texture of the hair very much, if possible.
- The application of the color must be professionally designed for the hair and adhered to every step of the way. (ShamBOOsie's Methodology)

Coloring, blending, or enhancing gray hair can be very difficult or very easy, depending on how much you know about gray hair. In the hair care business we measure the percentage of gray hair as *less than 25 percent, more than 25 percent, and 50 percent and above*, and *100 percent*. The method of coloring or covering is determined by the percentage of gray. If you have less than 25 percent gray, and it is scattered equally throughout the head, a semi-permanent color will work in most cases. When properly applied, semi-permanent color will last about three weeks or two shampoos. Many black hair salons use a temporary color for this purpose; many times this last only a few days, a week, and sometimes, if handled by an amateur, it may not take at all.

When working with 50 percent to 100 percent white and gray hair, this will be a full-time job. The white and gray strands will return and can be seen in as little as a week. It will be very tedious work when you have to Chemically Relax the hair every six to eight weeks and color the the New Growth on about the same schedule at two-week intervals. I suggest you wear a wig. Your hair will not be able to withstand the chemistry of the two chemicals applied repeatedly.

The Color of Hair

Hair is made mostly of protein also known as *keratin*. When hair is in its most healthy condition, it reflects light, causing the hair to shine. The pigmentation, which is actually the color in the hair, remains your natural hair color until you or someone else does something to alter the hair's natural color. White or gray hair has no color. The art of coloring the hair involves artificially changing the natural hair color/pigmentation of the hair. Since gray or white hair has no pigmentation, oftentimes the hair will be very resistant which means it will be more difficult to color.

There are a few important things to keep in mind when doing hair color at home: the *warmth* and *coolness* of a color, *tonality,* and most importantly, the *contributing pigment* (colors that are hidden in hair's natural pigmentation). Most of the hair colors you will probably use will fall within the *warmness* hair color, these will contain the colors of *red, yellow, orange, or gold* mixed within the overall formula. The *coolness* of a color will *contain blue, green, or violet.* Then there is the color *neutral* whose base is also *neutral.* These colors both warm and cool are called *base colors.* One or more of them can be found in all permanent hair color. They are hidden in the formula and listed on the packaging of permanent hair color.

Color Tip:

To keep things simple, when choosing a bottle of hair color, select one that has a base color of red, yellow, orange and red/violet (which will add a "wine flavor" to the mix) and of whatever shade and level you desire. Try to stay in the brown family of colors or medium and dark blond. If you should decide to go levels eight, nine, or ten, which are light, very light, and lightest blond, kiss your hair good-bye! Always keep a gold base in the mix, when you select a color, it will say so on the back of the package. These shades will be better for your complexion no matter what it is. These are the better shades for "Brown Beautiful Ladies."

Red-based color in brown tones (medium and light brown) will always create beautiful warm browns. If you choose a brown tone that doesn't have a red base, purchase a bottle of red hair color and add one-quarter ounce to the formula to achieve a lovely, soft, warm brown. Permanent red hair colors are in a family of their own. However, the base color is also red. Base colors are hidden in the overall coloring product and give a warm appearance to the color. The natural hair color of most black women is level one-black, level two-dark brown, or level three-light brown. To change your color another six shades to try and become blond, will destroy your hair.

Color Tip: Level one-Black as it applies to people of color is actually *Darkest Brown*. Knowing this will come in handy later in this chapter.

Color Tip:

When semi-permanent red and red/violet color (which only coats the hair shaft) is added to those natural brown colors, the result will be some of the most beautiful tones such as *Burgundy*, or *Mahogany*, and many lovely shades of reddish/brown that are perfect for brown skin tones.

Using Two Chemicals: This may sometimes be necessary. If properly applied, the *double chemical process* can be a beautiful styling concept. However, certain precautions must be taken. If you want to change your natural color to a darker shade, it will be easy enough for you to do at home. If you need a retouch or a virgin application, going lighter more than two levels, have the work done professionally. There are certain hidden color issues that only a Master Colorist would be aware of and be able to address. It is not advisable to attempt the work yourself.

Color Tip:

If you have attempted to do your own color and have "made a mess of things," don't try to fix it yourself, see a professional colorist.

Color Tip:

Permanent Hair color that doesn't contain Ammonia is a very important product improvement, especially for Chemically Relaxed hair. When you have *a Relaxer* in your hair and you need to use a permanent hair color perhaps for covering your gray, choose a permanent color that has very little or **"No Ammonia"** and use only a ten or twenty-volume developer.

Ammonia in hair color causes the hair to become very dry and porous after the service. The removal or reduction of ammonia has made permanent hair color for chemically relaxed hair much safer. An assortment of conditioners such as aloe vera, moisturizers, vitamins, and jojoba oil have been added to help strengthen and keep the hair moist and soft, after the service.

These colors are new on the market and have a much less drying effect on the hair. Women of color can now chemically relax and permanently color their hair while leaving the hair in a much better and healthier condition than ever before.

Color Tip:

Remember to allow at least seven full days and one shampoo and conditioner between the two processes.

Developers are sold in four different strengths—ten-, twenty-, thirty-, and forty-volume. One of the major mistakes people, including Hair Dressers will make is thinking developers are all the same, and peroxide is peroxide. This way of thinking will destroy your hair. Unless you intend to lighten the shade or tone of your hair one, two, or three levels, anything higher than twenty-volume developer will never be necessary. The numbers represents the level of change the coloring products will cause to your hair.

Color Tip:
Never use forty-volume developer on chemically relaxed hair. The damage to your hair will be extreme!

Color Tip:
If you want to color and lighten the shade of your hair only one level, when your natural color is black (level one), mix two ounces of ten-volume developer with two ounces of a color and shade of your choice, but the color should be one or two levels lighter than your natural hair color. A ten-volume developer will be gentler and will still result in a subtle change.

Because your hair is naturally very dark, changing it to a shade two, three, or four levels lighter normally would require a twenty- or thirty-volume developer, which is harsher on hair that has been chemically relaxed. It is best to use a lighter shade of color rather than a higher volume of developer.

Color Tip:
To go two, three, or four levels lighter, use twenty-volume developer. Choose a color and a shade you like, but one that is one or two levels lighter than you want to be. Do a *strand test* first, and time every stage of the process.

To do a *strand test,* select a small patch or section of hair and apply some of the same formula you will be using when you actually color your hair and start a half-inch from the scalp. Set a timer for thirty minutes and check the hair every five minutes. You can use up to forty-five minutes for this strand test, but the color should be removed as soon as you attain the desired color. Make a note of the time because it is the same amount of time that will be required for the rest of your hair. The timing should start after the color is applied, not before.

Color Tip:

It is not advisable to change the color of your hair more than three levels lighter than its natural shade. But if you must, it will require only a twenty-volume developer, as opposed to a thirty-volume developer, which will be milder and easier on your hair. For a subtle, gentle change of just one level, ten-volume will do the job and is always better.

The retouch of both the chemical relaxer and the permanent hair color must be restricted to the new growth only each time both processes are necessary. In this case, all the work should be done by a professional. There will be irreversible changes in the texture of the hair. A high quality shampoo and conditioner every four or five days should care very well for your hair.

Very Important:

Permanent Hair color is not designed for lightening natural color of your hair; this is a job for bleach or a lightener. It will lift your natural hair color, but it also deposits color at the same time. Permanent hair color is not designed for removing artificial hair color from your hair. Artificial, permanent or semi-permanent color can be removed with a color remover, an uncolor or a lightener/bleach. If the color is semi-permanent, use an uncolor designed for removal of semi-permanent hair color and a permanent color remover for permanent hair color.

Danger: Do Not Enter

This is the best way to begin telling you about the use of bleach, now referred to as a *lightener.*

The Essential Hair Loss Equation: Curly perm + Bleach =Hair Loss. Relaxer + Bleach = Hair Loss. Your Hair + Bleach = Hair Loss. The reason is because bleach eats away at everything that is left in the hair after it has it has been permed and relaxed and it leaves the hair with a cottonlike texture. People often tell me I look like the late singer Isaac Hayes because of the bald heads. If you ever use bleach and NO LYE RELAXER Kit in your hair, they will be telling you, too, that you look like Isaac Hayes & ShamBOOsie.

Color Tip:

This cotton-like change in the texture of your hair will be irreversible. It's practically impossible to stop the breakage, no matter what you use. My advice is to stay away from bleach altogether. (If you DO NOT use a relaxer in your hair, you may be able to get away with the use of bleach but condition well).

The texture of your hair must be strong enough to support a Perm (Thio) or a Relaxer (Sodium or No-Lye), and a Peroxide/ Ammonia base Permanent Hair color. All of these will have a softening effect on your hair shaft, which means it will become even more porous when permanent hair color is applied. For some hair textures this can be disastrous, while others can handle it with ease.

Other factors to be considered are:

- The level of color change.
- The strength of the peroxide.
- The length of time the color stays in the hair.
- The condition of the hair itself.
- The training of the person performing the service.

Relaxers (Sodium/Lye and No-Lye) and Hair color will create a much different effect. A Conditioning Sodium/Lye relaxer has a smooth, silky, hardening effect on the hair shaft, but will also leave the hair porous. The No-Lye relaxer has a rough, very drying effect on the hair, and it locks out or prevents moisture from entering the hair. Your hair is naturally dry, and when permanent hair color is added to the mix, it becomes even drier.

The Solution: You will need a thorough knowledge of the different types of hair color and conditioners that are available if you ever intend to color at home. It will be necessary to learn the proper way to use them to get the best results. This will be the secret to your success.

What is *Semi-permanent hair color?* Beautiful Browns, Jazzing, colored mousses, and many other types simply coat the hair shaft or penetrate slightly. When applied properly they can last two to four shampoos. There is also semi-permanent hair color and long lasting semi-permanent hair color, which are mixed with ten-volume peroxide and will last up to twenty-four shampoos, if you shampoo and condition your hair often.

- **What should you consider when choosing a hair color?**
- The color presently in the hair
- Your natural shade
- Your skin tone

- Your eye color
- Your age
- Your occupation
- The current condition of your hair
- **What are some of the better shades for women of color?**
- Gold, Warm Browns, Blond, and Auburn shades, colors containing some Reds, Dark Brown, Black, and Blue Black are well suited to brown skin tones.
- **Curls, Hair color, Relaxers, which will do the most damage?**
- When these products are used as directed, the level of change and damage to your hair texture will be minimal, in most cases, about the same for all three. Significant damage is caused by misuse or by error in formulation, application, and processing.
- **Should you color your gray and if so, what is the best way?**
- Yes, color it, if you desire. If the gray is greater than 50 percent and you are staying with your natural shade, use a *permanent hair color* with a ten or twenty-volume developer for the best results. If the gray is less than 25 percent, use a *long-lasting semi-permanent hair color* with a ten-volume developer.

Color Tip: If you like gray hair, there are products available for blending gray or enhancing gray to look beautiful. Check out Textures and Tones, and remember the better quality the product, the better the results.

- **"Will the amount and length of my hair make a difference when coloring my hair?"** Yes, it definitely will make a difference. Color works best when the hair is saturated which means that as much as two bottles of hair color, four ounces may be needed to do the job. This will become eight full ounces when mixed with four ounces of peroxide.

- Also if the hair is long, the ends of the hair have been around longer and are very porous. Therefore, the new growth, the middle, and the ends will have to be handled separately; I advise seeing a professional. If you have had color before and are getting a retouch, you could need two different formulas: one *permanent color* for the new growth and the other a *semi-permanent color* for the middle of the shaft and the ends of your hair.

- **"Should I shampoo my hair before I color it?"** It depends on the type of color you are using. It is all right to shampoo if you are using *temporary* or *semi-permanent* hair color. These are coaters, water-base colors and will disappear with the first shampoo. However, do not shampoo your hair if you are using a *long lasting semi-permanent* or a *permanent hair color*. This is because a developer is part of the formula and should only be applied to dry hair.

Except for *temporary* and *semi-permanent color*, you should always shampoo, but delay conditioning until you finish coloring. If the hair is oily or there is a buildup on the hair shaft, a clarifying shampoo, which is designed specifically for deep cleansing, may be needed. Remember to be very gentle when massaging the scalp and allow a couple of days between the shampoo and the use of *permanent hair color*.

Color Tip:

Always read the directions completely, before you start the application. You should do the same with every hair care product you intend to use on your hair.

- **"I have heard so much about the strand test, why is it important?"**
- This is one of the most important things you can do before coloring, because it is the surest way to know the end result before you

color your hair. If you were to use the same color as a friend, your color, in most cases, would turn out a different color.

- The reason is that no two people have the same natural color hair. The only time the hair will turn out the same is if you going darker. Remember, there are some hidden colors in your hair that will surprise you, if you are not aware they are there. These are called *contributing pigments*. Do a strand test to determine the appropriate timing to predict an accurate result.

- **"Will my hair type (straight, curly, dry, or oily, coarse or fine) change the time it will take to color my hair?"** Yes. Coarse hair will take longer for the color to penetrate. With medium and fine hair it is much faster. Whether the hair is straight, curly, or oily makes no difference.

- **"What is double processing?"**

- If the color you desire requires lifting your natural color two or three shades lighter, toning to achieve the desired shade is called *a double process*. In addition, anytime there is a chemical already in the hair, the addition of another chemical is *double processing*. If you have three chemicals in the hair this is called *triple processing*. Triple processing is never recommended.

- First the hair is lightened with a bleach or *lightener*. The toner is applied to give the hair its desired shade. This process will require a professional because the chosen toner must have the exact base color, which is found on every bottle of permanent hair color. To understand how to choose and use the base color will require the expertise of a professional colorist.

- There are basically two methods of applying *permanent hair color*: a Retouch and a Virgin method.

Homework: retouch method

You will need a willing friend to do the application; do not try this yourself. If you want to do the work at home, here is the correct way.

Remember to *always apply permanent hair color to dry hair.* Separate and clip the hair up into four sections, parting the hair down the center, and from ear to ear.

- Start in the back of the head with the first section and outline the section with hair color, to the new growth only. Make one-quarter inch horizontal partings and again apply the formula only to the new growth. Process until the desired shade is achieved or the allotted time. Rinse, shampoo, condition, and style. To refresh the middle of the shaft and ends of the hair, the color can be combed through the last five minutes of the process, but you must accurately time the entire process.

Color Tip:

Let me warn you, this is not something you want to try, unless some else is doing the work and you are the subject.

A virgin method means the hair has never been permanently colored before. Heat exits your body mostly through your scalp, and body heat plays an important role during the process of a virgin application. If the natural color of the hair is to be lightened, and heat is added to the mix, it speeds up the action of the hair color. One of the biggest mistakes people make, including many hairstylists, is to apply the color from the scalp through to the end of the hair.

Hot Roots:

I don't know if you are aware of this, but my mother use to tell me that the heat of the body escapes through the scalp. When I shave my head every other day, I will use warm soapy water, as soapy as possible. The body heat at the scalp causes the first half-inch of the hair closest to the scalp to lighten much faster lighter than the rest of the hair. This is called *hot roots,* and the result is that the hair will have two shades. The scalp area will look like it's "on fire." Correcting this can be tricky at best, and will require the knowhow of an expert colorist.

Virgin method:

Here is the correct way if you are going to lighten the hair, again, get a helper and remember to *always apply permanent hair color to dry hair.* Separate and clip the hair up into four sections. Starting in the back of the head, make one-quarter horizontal partings.

Apply plenty of color, starting one-half inch from the scalp and going all the way to the ends of the hair. After you have applied hair color to all sections, set a timer for twenty minutes. Next, apply color to the one-half inch at the scalp. When color is applied to all sections, set a timer and process up to forty-five minutes, this will include the first twenty minutes.

Color Tip:

The term *"up to"* means use as much time as you need which is not always forty-five minutes, but never more than forty-five minutes.

Virgin method with a darker color: Apply the hair color from the scalp to the ends of the hair. If you are using a *temporary, semi-permanent, or a long lasting semi-permanent hair color,* use this same method of application. Process the allotted time; rinse until the water runs clear.

Color Tip:

Do Not shampoo your hair. Condition and style as usual.

How to neutralize unwanted colors:

Listed below are colors that will neutralize each other.

- Red + Green
- Yellow + Violet
- Orange + Blue
- Red Orange + Blue Green
- Yellow Orange + Blue Violet
- Yellow Green + Red Violet

Now, what does all this mean?

Let's say you have colored your hair, and it turned out to be redder than you wanted. To get rid of the red or tone it down, purchase another color similar to the shade you used but with a base color of green. As you remember, we learned previously that green neutralizes red and just the opposite. Follow this same principle when dealing with every other unwanted color. The base color is always listed on the bottle, just below the primary shade. Another way to deal with unwanted colors is to formulate the color that will neutralize the unwanted color. These are called secondary colors.

- Yellow + Red = Orange
- Red +Blue = Violet
- Blue + Yellow = Green

If, for some reason, the hair turns out green or greenish, apply red for just five minutes. If it turns out yellow or gold, apply red mixed with blue to make violet, which will neutralize the gold or yellow tones. Use the same principles to deal with every other unwanted color. This system will work whether the hair color is *permanent, semi-permanent,* or *temporary.*

The Tale of Scary Red

A client, Sonia, came in with bright red hair and said she couldn't stand to look at it another day. I lightly shampooed her hair. I then mixed blue and yellow, which made the most beautiful green hair color I have ever seen. I showed it to Sonia and said, "This will do the trick." Well, I thought she would pass out from the thought of possibly having green hair!

It took me some time to talk her into trusting me to put this green hair color on her hair. Finally, after much coaxing, she allowed me to apply the green hair color to her hair. I let it sit for a few minutes. As I checked to see if it was working, I made these awful facial grimaces, which caused Sonia much concern. (Of course, I knew this client very well, and knew that she was good hearted and could take a joke.)

After about five minutes I rinsed, shampooed, and conditioned her hair. I was careful not to allow her to see the final result, which drove her crazy, and I loved every minute of it! Finally, she looked in the mirror, and (with a sign of relief) what she saw was a beautiful warm brown! (We have laughed about this during her many subsequent visits to the salon.)

Bob Barker, the star of the *The Price is Right* colored his hair well into his late sixties. In order to color so often, one would have to on occasion have all of the color removed and reapplied or the hair could get very dark from too many applications by absorbing too much color during each retouch. Bob Barker tells the story that one day while he was having his color removed; he received a call from his producers telling him that one of the shows had to be retaped. He was told that the shooting could not wait. At the time, his hair was white, and no one had ever seen him with white hair. When he walked on stage to reshoot the show, the audience gave him a standing ovation. They loved it! Needless to say, Bob Barker didn't color his hair anymore after that.

The higher the percentage of gray, the more work your hair will have to have to do to cover or color it. This is the reason temporary and semi-permanent hair color does not cover the gray hair very well when the percentage of gray is greater than twenty-five. The question is how you can use permanent hair color safely while wearing a relaxer? Today you no longer have to settle for basic black, you can wear any color or any mixture of colors you desire.

Gray hair has no pigmentation (color) and can be very resistant and very difficult to color because the color solution will not penetrate the hair shaft. If the hair is also coarse, it can add to the problem of coloring the hair. If this is the case, you may want to presoften the hair with two ounces of a neutral color and two ounces of two-volume developer.

Process for about twenty minutes, and then apply the color formula you have chosen for your hair, and process up to forty-five minutes. Check the hair after twenty minutes, then every five minutes. Remove the formula as soon as the hair is ready.

You may also start out by increasing the developer to thirty-volume, use a shade one level lighter in color, and process up to forty-five minutes. Check after twenty minutes, and then every five minutes.

Color Tip:
Use the amount of time you need, but do not exceed forty-five minutes.

Remember there is an assortment of hair colors available that can also be mixed to formulate something quite lovely for your hair. However you mix or formulate them, be sure to keep an exact record for future reference.

Beautiful Black Hair

You'll Wonder Where the Yellow Went

You can be sure that when the hair is pretty and white it will get dirty and turn yellow.

I can still remember seeing the little old ladies in church with blue hair when I was a young boy. This was the result of misuse of a product that was designed to remove the yellow from their gray hair. Yellow in gray hair can be caused by a number of things. It can be due to a buildup of styling aids, such as hair sprays and spritz. It can be due to smoking, dirty hot irons, medication, or from lack of proper shampooing and conditioning.

Color Tip:

Choose a clear hair color, mix two ounces with two ounces of ten-volume developer and apply it to dry hair, process for twenty-five minutes, rinse, shampoo, condition, and style.

There are many ways to neutralize yellow anywhere you find it. There are many products on the market that are made especially for removing yellow. You want to choose the one perfect for your hair. Always, with every product you buy and use on your hair, read all of the manufacturer's suggestions and directions, very slowly and very carefully before you apply them.

ShamBOOsie Suggests *The Beautiful Collection,* which is a gentle, cream permanent hair color made especially for use on chemically relaxed hair. Clairol Professional researched and designed a color system made especially with you in mind. They removed most of the ammonia normally found in *permanent hair color.*

The pH scale:

Everything we use on or in our hair is a chemical, including water, and is measured on what is called a pH scale, which is a symbol for

216

potential hydrogen concentration, which is the degree of acidity or alkalinity in a product. The pH scale goes from 0 to 14, with 7 being the balancing point. Everything to the left of 7 is acid, and everything to the right is alkaline.

The closer a product is to 1, the stronger it is on the acid side, and the closer a product is to 14 the stronger it is on the alkaline side. The difference in the types of shampoos and the factor to be considered when selecting a shampoo is whether it is *pH balanced*. The one you should use is about 4.5 on the pH scale.

A List pH values:

- Color rinses 2.5
- Vinegar 2.7
- Neutralizers 3.0
- Hair 4.5 to 5.0
- Skin 4.5 to 6.0
- Shampoo (for your hair type) 4.0 to 4.5
- Water 7
- Blood 7.3
- Stronger shampoos 7.0 to 10.0
- Water softeners 10.5
- Hair straighteners 11.0
- Ammonia 11.8
- Bleach or lighteners 12.0 to 14
- Lye Relaxers 14
- No-Lye Relaxers 14.0 to around 18.0, off the scale

When we chemically relax hair with a **Conditioning Lye Relaxer**, it shoots up very high on the *pH scale*. Neutralization will bring the pH back down, and normalize the hair around 8.5 and 7.0 by the middle of the week. So the hair needs the time to return to 7.0, and it will need a very good shampoo and conditioner before permanently coloring the hair, a week later.

This theory is closely associated with the reason the **No-Lye Relaxer** is so dangerous. When we chemically relax the hair with a **No-Lye Relaxer**, once again the hair shoots up very high on the *pH scale*. Neutralization, in this case, will stop the action of the chemical, but does not lower the pH, leaving the hair very high on the *pH scale*, which causes calcium build up.

Color Tip:

When the hair is blow dried for styling, it becomes very hard to the touch, brittle, and will inevitably break and shed quickly. Add *permanent hair color* to the mix and "have yourself a bald!"

Good luck and Color your world with hope of GROW-ING lovely hair!

Chapter 11

Master the Art of Applying a Chemical "LYE" Relaxer

Every black female must **Master the Art of Applying A Chemical "LYE" Relaxer** like she learns to cook and make her own clothing. She must teach her daughters to **Master the Art of Applying A Chemical "LYE" Relaxer!** It is **ShamBOOsie's** intension to teach **every black female** in the country how to apply this Chemical, but to **NEVER Self-Apply this Chemical.** There MUST always be two people involved—one applying the Chemical and the other receiving the Chemical application! Black women you can put an end to your struggle with this most unusually difficult hair, and **STOP** giving away **$9 billion** every year the very moment you **Master the Art of Applying a Chemical LYE Relaxer!** The **No-Scalp Burn** application technique developed by **ShamBOOsie** is very simple, and anyone can learn it!

You have been applying this mysterious Chemical the **Wrong Way!** You will continue to lose your hair, and your daughters will never **GROW** their hair longer than two to three inches, until you take the time to **Master the Art of Applying a Chemical LYE Relaxer!** Then you should teach it to every female and every male in your family!

Beautiful Black Hair

Use of the **Chemical No-Lye Relaxer Kit** will destroy your hair every time it's applied because of the **DRYNESS** it causes. This **DRYNESS** is the reason so many **Black Women** and their **Daughters** have badly damaged broken hair! The manufacturers will continue to take your money until you find the time to watch the **DVD**, read this book from **cover to cover,** and practice the application method until you have **Mastered the Art of Applying a Chemical LYE Relaxer!**

Next you must Master the Art of selecting and applying/using Conditioners and Shampoos. The key to sustaining your hair is knowing the perfect Conditioners to use on Chemically Relaxed hair. It is the Mastering of these two application techniques that will change your life forever. Your HAIR will **GROW and GROW and GROW!** (I recommend that you ALWAYS have your Chemical Relaxers applied buy a professional, in a salon setting. Remember, **"It Takes two Baby—Me and You. It takes two!)** **Meaning don't Self-Apply a relaxer kit or any other type of chemical!**

Here is Another Possibility!

When you master these techniques, you will be able to apply this Chemical and make plenty of money in your neighborhood. It is not my intention to cut out the middle man, the Hairdresser, but **I** believe that if someone or many manufacturers are going to continue and create a "Chemical No-LYE Relaxer Kit" and put this Trick in a Box on store shelves for you to apply, **ShamBOOsie** MUST teach every black female how the application process WORKS!

Every Black Female Must Learn to Apply this Chemical!

The majority of the hair care issues the black woman has with her hair can be solved by learning all there is to know about her hair and how to care for it!

You must learn the proper way to apply the Chemical LYE Relaxer. The problem has always been Scalp Burns and ShamBOOsie has taken care of this problem! There is no way to "Self-Apply" a Chemical "LYE" Relaxer and keep the hair in place. The hair will eventually break and fall out from being so weakened by combing the Chemical through the hair repeatedly. This very thin, very fine hair fiber cannot withstand the combing of such a Chemical through it over and over again.

However, this is only one of the many problems incurred from combing a chemical through the hair repeatedly. Remember, the very application of a Calcium Hydroxide Chemical "No-LYE" Relaxer Kit will cause the hair to become so excessively dry that the hair will "SNAP" "CRACKLE," and "POP" until there is no hair left on the head. This is costing black women collectively $9 billion each year, and all of that money is going into the hands of people that could care less if your hair falls out! I cannot say enough to stress how destructive this Chemical truly is.

The only solution that makes sense is to become so skilled in applying the Chemical "LYE" Relaxer that you will be able to do this without causing scalp burns ever! This is exactly what I am hoping to teach every black female on the planet; it is possible if each black female in every family would find the time to learn this most important process. As long as black women continue to allow the manufacturers to dictate how they handle the application of the relaxer and more importantly, as long as they continue to use the Calcium Hydroxide Chemical "No-LYE" Relaxer Kit, they will continue to lose her hair and throw away $9 billion a year. Don't settle for having your hair fall out repeatedly, year after year.

You must nail down all there is to know about this Chemical such as:

- How this Chemical really works
- How to apply the Chemical
- Where the Chemical should be applied (New Growth only)
- How long to leave the Chemical on the hair
- Where to begin applying the Chemical
- When to remove the Chemical
- How to remove the Chemical; which sections to remove first
- Applying the relaxer is a time-sensitive process

What is left is the selection of the proper Conditioners and Shampoos, then learning how to use the right kinds of conditioner and shampoos. You MUST learn what a Conditioner is, how Shampoos work, and which ones are best to use for black hair and Chemically Relaxed Hair. You MUST understand that it is the Conditioners and Shampoos that keep the hair Strong, keep it Soft to Touch, Keep it GROWING, and Stop it from Breaking. Conditioners and Shampoos also Relieve or Reverse DRYNESS, give the hair body and bounce, and help hair hold curls and even a bend in the hair. If you learn how Conditioners and Shampoos work, it will completely change everything with your hair.

You MUST understand what a "Calcium Hydroxide" Chemical "No-LYE" Relaxer Kit does to your hair. The same is true with the application of every other product, including shampoo, oils of every kind, hair sprays, gels, crèmes, liquids, hair color, bleach or lighteners, and even temporary colors and water.

If you are going to apply a Chemical Relaxer to your own hair, ask this question: "How will this Chemical straighten my hair?" If you can't answer this question, you may not want to apply this Chemical to your hair.

The Chemical LYE Relaxer is by far the BEST Chemical Relaxer ever created for the purpose of relaxing hair! **Everyone has been** applying this mysterious Chemical the **Wrong Way** and 100 or 1,000 women will apply this Chemical 100 and 1,000 different ways because everyone is guessing! You will continue to lose your hair and your daughters will never **GROW** their hair longer than two or three inches, until someone takes the time to **Master the Art of Applying a Chemical "LYE" Relaxer!**

When you learn to select the PERFECT Conditioners and Shampoos, you will be able to really condition your hair because the LYE Relaxer allows the hair to still have the ability to receive the nourishing properties found in High-End Conditioners and Shampoos. After applying a **Chemical No LYE Relaxer Kit,** the extreme **DRYNESS BLOCKS and LOCKS OUT** the hair's ability to receive the nourishing properties found in High-End, Conditioners and Shampoos. Conditioners hold the hair together, softly but strongly and never dry OUT the hair; DRYNESS = BREAKAGE! Reversing the DRYNESS Stops the Breakage. The No-LYE Relaxer is designed to cause damage, dry out your hair, cause it to break, and get you to spend more of your hard earned money.

ShamBOOsie has perfected the "Hair Wellness Approach" to applying a **Chemical LYE Relaxer.** I have made it so simple that you can learn everything an hour or so. You should practice using any kind of inexpensive white crème! Buy and use a jar of cheap Conditioner instead of your Chemical Relaxer, to practice the chemical application. You will be able to rinse the conditioner and you can practice the process again and again if necessary to get it right.

This is a simple application method that you will only have to learn once. It will not take long for you and your daughters to GROW hair shoulder length or longer. It is my hope that "each one will teach one" because this process really works. It is a "see and do" process. Just practice exactly what you see and do not change the process. **Use ONLY a Conditioning LYE Relaxer** when the real application process starts! You MUST apply and remove the Chemical in a timely fashion, using the exact outlined method. This is the reason I ask you to read the entire book, from cover to cover!

This process WORKS! This is the way your hair truly works. This book is scientifically correct so the reader never has to make the wrong decision when selecting and applying a chemical. You will select the best Conditioners and Shampoos, which are the most important products you will need to always have on hand. **Dudley's Products** is the only hair care line manufactured by black people that **ShamBOOsie** will use. Their full line is High-End and is great as long as there *is not* a **NO-LYE RELAXER** in the hair. Where there *is* a **No-LYE Relaxer Kit** in the hair, ONLY **Humectress Moisturizing Conditioner** and **Therappe Shampoo from Nexxus Products** will aid in reversing the extreme DRYNESS and Hair Breakage. You will also need **Crème Press Hairdressing** from Dudley's Products.

If you should ever GROW your hair down your back, which I truly believe is possible for most black women, you have to convince yourself that you are getting ready to do the work needed to make your hair more beautiful than ever before. You may remember also that all High-End Hair Care Products are made well and will work for you.

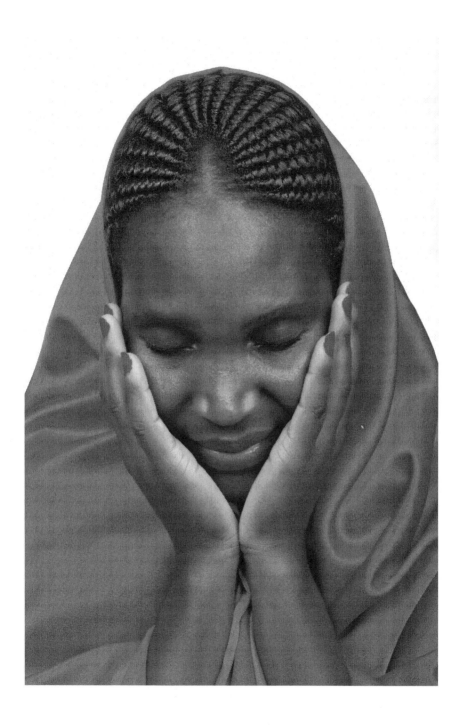

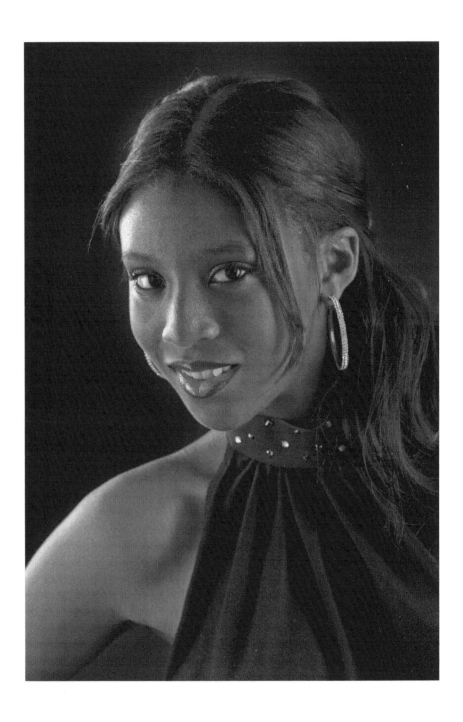

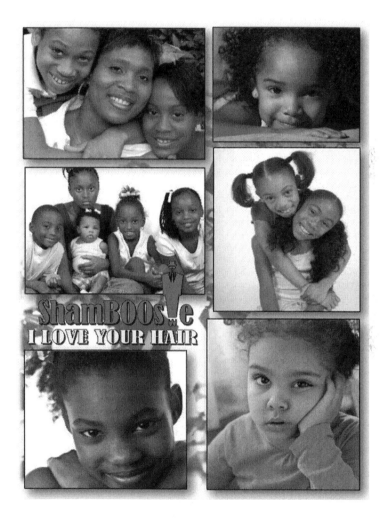

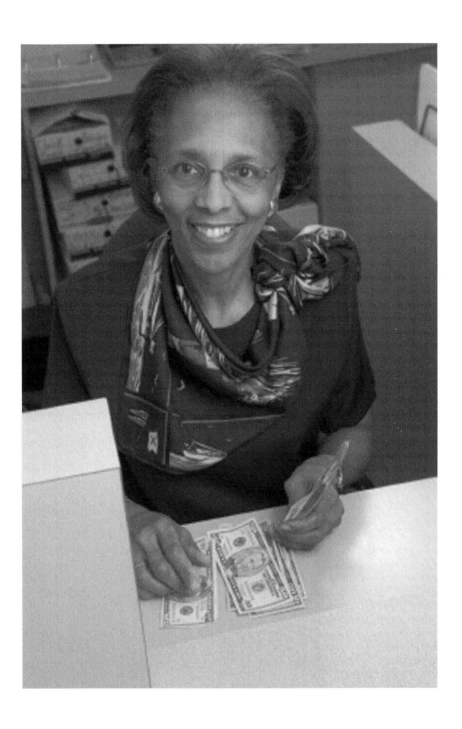

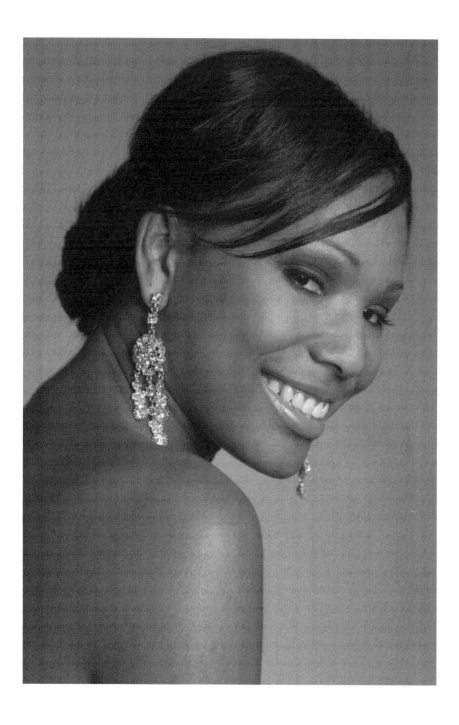

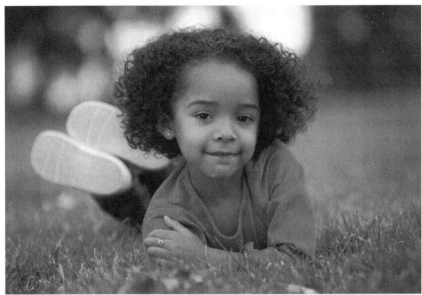

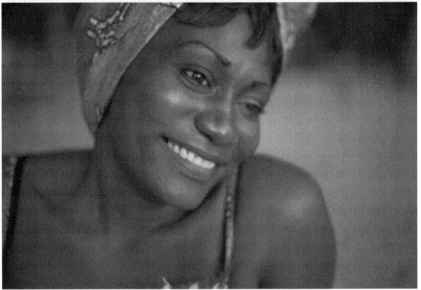

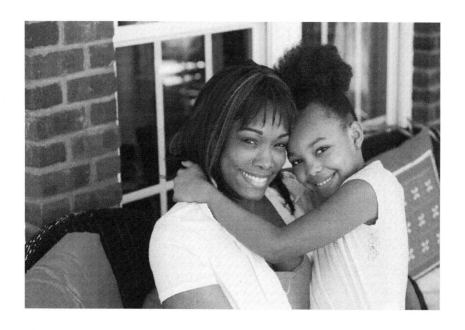

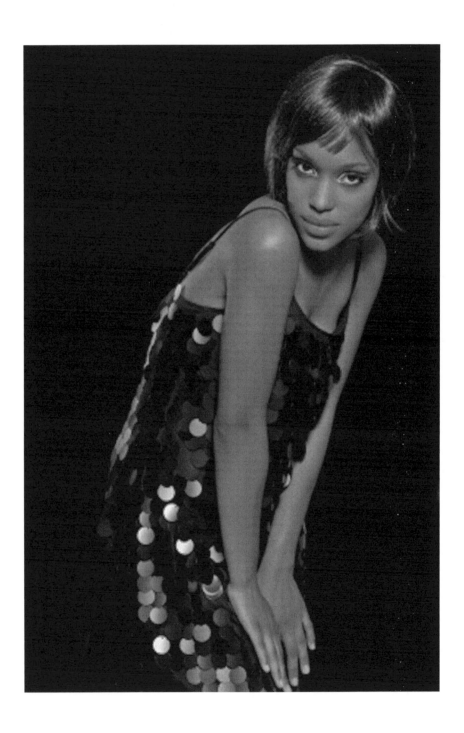

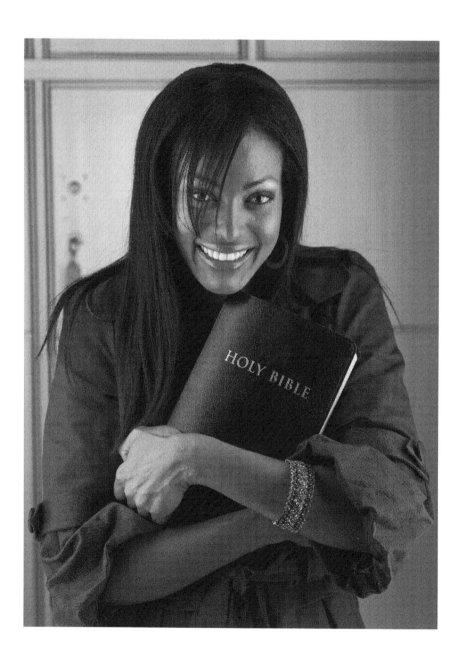

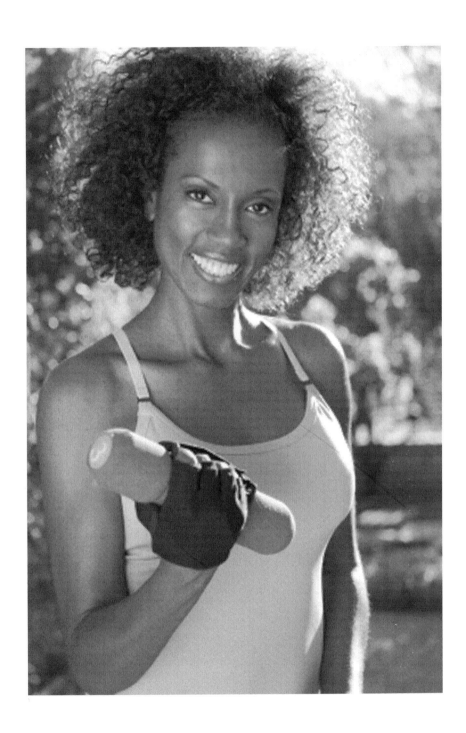

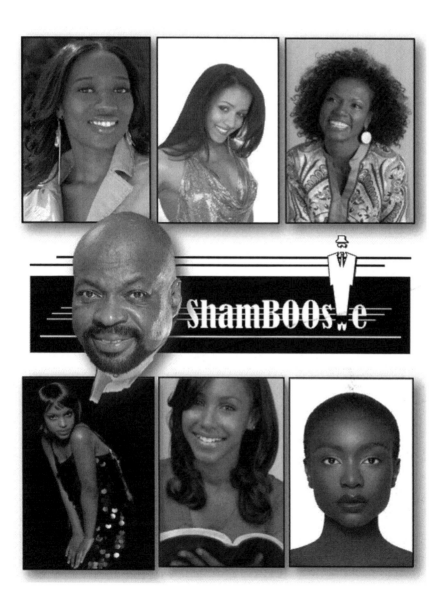

Chapter 12

The Chemical No LYE Relaxer Kit: A Trick in a BOX!

A Chemical but NOT a Relaxer; It's a Silent Man-made Dehydrating Hair Destroyer—DEHYDRATING MONSTER.

Because of **The Chemical No-LYE Relaxer Kit, manufacturers have black women Going in Circles!** They are purchasing cheap, poor quality hair products, and **the Chemical No-LYE Relaxer Kit.** (I can't even call them hair CARE products). This is one scheme that affects every black female in America; **Product Manufacturers** are selling Chemicals they know will DRY OUT and take OUT your HAIR. These poor quality products include shampoos, conditioners, and oils that do nothing for your hair except ensure that it will fall out! Also, their Styling Sprays cause even more DRYNESS because of their alcohol content! Then in six to eight weeks over twenty million black females around the country, start the whole process over again—**the BREAKAGE never STOPS!**

The Korean Distributors on the other hand have no idea of what they are selling and don't really care. **The Koreans** have found a"

Beautiful Black Hair

Gold Mine" in the black community. They distribute 80 percent of all the black hair products sold in America. They have also set up their own stores in black communities and ship their cheap goods ONLY to their stores. They sell about 85 percent of all the FALSE HAIR black women are using.

It Is Amazing How Dry the Hair Really Gets and Why!

It is the continuous use of the **Chemical No-LYE Relaxer Kits** that causes the extreme dryness and breakage that threatens to leave you and your daughters bald.

There are different types of dryness in black hair.

- Black hair is normally dry by nature.
- Black hair becomes drier with the use of a **Lye Relaxer** but is manageable.
- Black hair becomes extremely dry with the use of a **No-Lye Relaxer** and prone to breakage.
- Permanent Hair Color and a **Lye Relaxer** will cause a different type of dryness in the hair, but it is manageable.
- The most dangerous form of dry hair is found in hair treated with a **No-Lye Relaxer** and the use of bleach.
- The second most dangerous form of dry hair is hair treated with a **No-Lye Relaxer** and permanent hair color.
- The worst kind of dryness in hair comes from using a No-Lye Relaxer Kit, permanent hair color with thirty-volume developer, and a concentrated hair conditioner. If there is a No-Lye Relaxer in your hair, then put in braids or a weave and wait six weeks and comb another No-Lye Relaxer through what is left of it. Then use cheap hair product to try and care for it. Oops! Welcome to **"Baldsville, USA."**

There Are Many Things Black Women Cannot Do to Their Hair

The Chemical Hair Relaxer is the one thing that relates to black women, but not to any race of Women whose hair GROWS straight. The very tight curls in black hair appear to be a curse, yet this very problematic hair can actually be managed with simplicity. The important factor is mastering the application of the Chemical Hair Relaxer every six to eight weeks.

The restriction of GROWTH of the black woman's hair is due mostly to what she allows to be done to her hair, and what she does to it herself. In a word, she is responsible for her hair and the totality of its health and GROWTH. **There are things a black woman cannot do as long as she wears a Chemical Relaxer!** If you insist, you will lose your hair and the manufacturers will love you for doing it.

- You cannot use a Chemical No-LYE Relaxer, your daughters cannot use a Chemical, and no one you know can use a Chemical No-LYE Relaxer, EVER! **Insist and Lose Your Hair.**
- You cannot Chemically Relax your hair and apply your own permanent hair color or allow an amateur to apply your color and Chemicals. **Insist and Lose Your Hair.**
- You cannot Chemical Relax your hair and apply your own Bleach or allow an amateur to apply your bleach. You cannot wear bleach and a Chemical Relaxer, LYE or No-LYE Relaxer. **Insist and Lose Your Hair.**
- You cannot wear a Chemical Relaxer and Hot Curl your hair every day! **Insist and Lose Your Hair.**
- You cannot wear a Chemical Relaxer and flat iron your hair every day! **Insist and Lose Your Hair.**
- You cannot wear a Chemical Relaxer and use poor quality, cheap Hair Care product! **Insist and Lose Your Hair.**

- You cannot wear a Chemical Relaxer and never use conditioners and shampoos. **Insist and Lose Your Hair.**
- You cannot wear a Chemical Relaxer and use cheap conditioners and shampoos. **Insist and Lose Your Hair.**
- You cannot wear a Chemical Relaxer and comb No-Lye Relaxer through your hair even once and keep your hair. **Insist and Lose You Your Hair.**
- You cannot Self-Apply a Chemical Relaxer and keep the hair. **Insist and Lose Your Hair.**
- You cannot wear a Chemical Relaxer and suddenly decide to STOP! **Insist and Lose Your Hair.**
- You cannot comb No-Lye Relaxer or any other type of Chemical Relaxer through your daughters' hair, until you learn how and Master the Art of Application! **Insist and she will Lose her Hair.**

The use of a **Chemical No-LYE Relaxer** changes everything! You must upgrade your Conditioners and Shampoos, and use light sheens that don't weight the hair down like heavy OILS. Use **Crème Press Hairdressing** and settle this thing with OIL once and for all! Once you discover what **Crème Press Hairdressing** is capable of, you will pray that Dudley's Products never stops making this miracle hairdressing. Take the time to learn how your hair WORKS! You can trust this book, and you can trust **ShamBOOsie.**

The Chemical No-LYE Relaxer Kit is **a trick in a box.** It promises hair like Rice Krispies **that snaps, crackles, and pops!** The women using these cheap chemicals and products are **"Kitchen Chemists"**- hairdressers without a license to practice.

Why do I teach ShamBOOsie's method of the Chemical LYE Relaxer (No Scalp Burn) Application? First I want to make sure my readers fully understand, that as a Professional Teacher of Hair techniques, and a licensed Hairdresser, I must recommend that you seek out a Professional Stylist for your **Conditioning LYE Relaxer** service. **The Lye Relaxer** does NOT come in a kit, thank God! It is very important that you NEVER allow anyone to apply a **Chemical NO-LYE Relaxer Kit** to your hair, unless you want to lose your hair. To **Self-Apply a Chemical NO-LYE Relaxer Kit** to your hair will be the biggest mistake you will ever make; don't allow anyone to tell you otherwise. You will lose all of your hair and very fast because of the extreme dryness **Chemical NO-LYE Relaxer Kit** will cause! A conditioning Lye Relaxer is a 1000 times better!

I know that finding someone who can safely apply your **Conditioning LYE Relaxer** will not be easy, and so the next best thing is for you to learn, really learn **ShamBOOsie's Hair Wellness Method of Application**. This will include learning as much as possible about the chemical, how it works when relaxing your hair, and how best to condition your hair before and after each Chemical Application. There are no Conditioners formulated to keep your hair as healthy as possible, and made available to you under the heading **black hair care products.**

You should also know that there is no such thing as "Black Hair Care Products!" It's a myth just like believing you can't GROW and have long, straight, flowing hair! This is very possible if you learn how to properly apply a Conditioning LYE Relaxer. **It is a two-person process!** You MUST learn how to apply the **Conditioning LYE Relaxer** and someone else must learn how to apply your **Conditioning LYE Relaxer. ShamBOOsie** will be the one to teach you ALL of the secrets to getting it right.

Beautiful Black Hair

ShamBOOsie's Wellness Approach Is Intensive Care for Your Hair

I have Designed and Created a method by which black women can Chemically Straighten their hair and GROW it Shoulder Length or Longer and the HAIR will remain Strong, soft to the touch, and healthy. **Now I need to get the word out!**

Your Damaged Hair Cannot be Repaired, It Must be Replaced with Newly Grown Hair! Nothing, not even GROWTH, is possible until you get complete control of the dryness in your hair. Controlling the dryness STOPS the breakage. This entire book is structured around the idea of GROWING new hair. It is why I spend so much time talking about the importance shampooing and CONDITIONING the hair often and on a regular basis. There is no way to avoid shampooing and conditioning your hair, if your intention is to keep the newly GROWN hair. You may feel that you don't have the time to condition your hair. However, your success will require a commitment to put everything in perspective as it relates to the overall health of your hair. There will be a need for change, adjustment, and sacrifice, but if you follow the plan, you will get the desired results. That's a promise!

The Chemical No-Lye Relaxer Kit is a **Dehydrating Monster in a box** that literally destroys the hair, yet this extremely destructive product remains on store shelves. Sadly, the product manufacturers are making billions of dollars in profits while black women are collectively spending $9 billion a year and losing their hair!

The victim is the black woman and her Hair! Many Hair Diseases are silent hair killers that totally degrade the hair fiber before the victim is able to find a line of hair care product capable of handling this **Dehydrating Monster!** There are no warning signs, only vague symptoms like the apparent and extreme DRYNESS that appears seemingly from out of nowhere. The ability to eliminate the dryness or slow the rate at which the hair is breaking and falling out seems impossible.

This **Dehydrating Monster** is a force of damage that has a will of its own! The hair will pop and break at will in short and long pieces, even full-length strands of your hair will come out. In the process of trying to get your Newly Grown hair straight, combing this very destructive Chemical through your hair, **The Chemical NO-LYE Relaxer Kit** doesn't really get the hair straight. Your hair ends up retaining unwanted curl that cannot be Chemically straightened or relaxed. The curl has been "locked in" the hair by something unknown. Even the best Hair Care Products appear to have little or no effect on this hair and many other problems created by the **Chemical NO-LYE Relaxer Kit.**

Regular visits to the salon to seek answers and early diagnosis from a hair consultant, usually bring unexplained or vague solutions, and a feeling that there are no real answers. She watches her hair deteriorating quickly before her eyes. As the damage becomes worse if it's not treated, she is not sure that she can save her hair or the very life of her hair because no one has ever made a hair product to address the many issues. Unfortunately, women continue using this very toxic, dangerous chemical, subconsciously thinking that it is safer. In reality, it is not. I repeat: **the No-Lye Relaxer Kit is not safe to** use! **It is a Dehydrating Monster!** This chemical is extremely dangerous and destroys hair.

The best and safest way to apply the **Chemical LYE Relaxer** at home is to learn how and to understand that it is a two-person process. But before anything else takes place, learn HOW! It will take twenty-four to thirty-six months to GROW out the damage left after using a **No-Lye (Calcium Hydroxide) Relaxer.** No Conditioner, Shampoo, Oil, or Moisturizer, regardless to price or quality level, will be able to reverse or even manage the damage that the **No-Lye Relaxer** will leave in the hair.

Even the Highest Quality of Hair Care Products on the market will not work! The only answer will be to GROW new hair to replace the damaged hair. Hair products are not formulated to address the problems caused by the **No-Lye Relaxer Kit**. Shame on L'Oreal and others that have joined in this money making venture! No one is making hair care products to address the problems with your hair, but instead many hair product companies are cashing in on your lack of knowledge. It's like taking your car to a mechanic to have it fixed, and the mechanic does something to your car that will cause you to return for more service. Except in this case, the black woman has to return for service every six to eight weeks!

The Makers of these chemicals know that using their **No-Lye Relaxer Kit** damages hair. Just look at the list of other products the company makes to address the problems. The hair is being damaged by using the **No-Lye Relaxer Kit** and by using cheap hair products that do nothing, and in six to eight weeks the process must be started all over again. It is like going in circles damaging the hair with every application. Once the hair is relaxed, it MUST continue to be relaxed or there will be hair loss. There is hair loss either way.

It's a Dehydrating Monster! One company makes a **No-Lye Relaxer** that promises "85 percent less breakage." This is like "promising 15 percent hair breakage! " They are actually saying that you will only lose 15 percent of your hair when you apply a **No-Lye Relaxer.** This has cost **Product Manufacturers** revenues of over $350 million. Now that **Product Manufacturers** have caused her to lose all of her hair and now that she has less of a reason to purchase their hair products because she has no hair; L'Oreal has made a new product to help her keep her weave healthy—a new FALSE HAIR care product.

Deceptions Beneath the Deception

First there is the DECEPTION that the No-Lye Relaxer is a Relaxer! No-Lye Relaxer is **NOT** a Relaxer and does NOT relax or straighten hair. But the greatest DECEPTION is the consumer's lack of knowledge about Chemical Relaxers. She doesn't know or understand the Chemistry of the many chemicals on the market, their chemical makeup, or the Chemistry of her hair. This disadvantage has provided **Manufacturers** with an advantage that has been worth billions over the past twenty-two or so years. **Product Manufacturers** are literally "BANKING" on the consumer never finding out all of the harm The **No-Lye Relaxer,** is causing. **There are so many unknowns.**

Other Deceptions

- She doesn't know that the very chemistry, formula, and makeup of this imposter, is her greatest threat of hair loss. **Using the No-Lye Relaxer causes her to have No Hair!** It is also the reason this chemical is **NOT** a Chemical Relaxer, as they claim.
- She doesn't know that **The No-Lye Relaxer Kit** causes BALDNESS!
- She doesn't know that just the application of this chemical guarantees her hair will fall out because of the makeup of the chemical. **Calcium Hydroxide (the chemical formula) dries excessively and causes breakage.** The self-application of combing this chemical through her hair repeatedly speeds up the hair loss process 100 percent. When she adds in the cheap maintenance conditioners, shampoos, and a long list of oily products that are supposed to keep the extreme dryness under control, but do not,

then she is "sitting in a donut hole," and getting ripped-off from every direction.

- This is not a chemical relaxer and is a product that should never be used on human hair!
- She doesn't know that this product is the "Most Damaging and Most Destructive" chemical the Industry has even created.
- She has no idea that this chemical forms a different type of curl in the hair that cannot ever be straightened or removed from the hair. Even combing the chemical through her hair will not work. No chemical, not even a **Lye Relaxer** will remove this curl from the hair because the No-Lye Relaxer has locked the curls in the hair, by destroying the natural bonds of the hair. It is the neutralization or the destroying of the natural bonds of her hair that is supposed to cause the chemical relaxer to straighten and relax the hair.
- Many of you get your hair relaxed only to find that somehow, the relaxer didn't take. The No-Lye Relaxer destroys the natural bonds of the hair and many times has locked unwanted the curl in the hair, preventing the hair from ever being relaxed straight which was the reason or purpose of "Self-Applying" the relaxer in the first place.
- She doesn't know how the relaxer will change the texture of the hair.
- She doesn't know that the No-Lye Relaxer really isn't a relaxer at all.
- She doesn't know that this chemical will leave her hair with curl that can never be removed from her hair, which means that once she uses a No-Lye Relaxer, she will never be able to get her hair to relax!
- She doesn't know that L'Oreal, the Koreans, and other white-owned companies are cashing in on her lack of knowledge big time!

- She doesn't know that this chemical will cause extreme, extraordinary dryness in her hair, causing it to fall out.
- She doesn't know that self-application will cause her hair to fall out!
- She doesn't know that combing the chemical through her hair repeatedly causes her hair to fall out, to stretch, and each strand becomes weaker and more susceptible to hair breakage.
- She doesn't know that trying to get her hair "bone straight" will not stop the new growth from returning.
- She doesn't know that cheap conditioners and shampoos don't work! So the hair doesn't really have anything to protect it and keep it healthy.
- She doesn't know that she should never "self-apply" any type of chemical relaxer. The conditioner is the most important product she will need, and must always have on hand. It must be the best!
- She doesn't know that she shouldn't apply this very dangerous No-Lye Relaxer even to her daughter's hair because it will cause her hair to fall out.
- She doesn't know that the No-Lye Relaxer was not created to work or to relax hair. Instead it was created to "trick" her into believing it was a new invention, and that No-Lye was safer than Lye relaxers. It was all a trick from the very beginning. A lie!
- If she uses a No-Lye Relaxer it will dry her hair out. Normally, the way most people attempt to strengthen damaged or weak hair is by treating the hair with a protein conditioner. When No-Lye Relaxer is in the hair, and has severely dried out, the hair, treating the hair with a concentrated protein conditioner intensifies the dryness and quadruples the chance for breakage.
- When her scalp itches badly and it is a sign that it's time for her dreaded relaxer that must be done every six to eight weeks, like it or not. However, she is relaxing her "New Growth" the wrong way. When she combs relaxer through hair, over and over,

it causes the hair to become fine, thin, weak, and extremely dry. She is causing her newly grown hair to fall out!

How is it possible that black women are collectively spending $9 billion on hair care annually? They are less than 10 percent of the population! Where are the billions coming from?

The Beauty Salon Business was once a viable source of income for black women until **Product Manufacturers** put the chemical relaxer in a box and placed it on store shelves for sale to the general public! A single black women that owned her own salon with four chairs could make 50 percent of all the work from three of the chairs and 100 percent of the money from her own chair. If her salon did exceptional work, the owner could clear over $150,000.00 and up to $300,000.00 a year. Her overhead was hair products, utilities, and rent on the building. In the early 1980s, "the curl" was very popular, and I did them for $90.00-$150.00 per customer. I called myself "the Curl King," but I was far from it. After three years in the business, I did a few $1,500.00 days. I trained a black woman who made $90,000.00 by the end of her second year, owning her own salon, and she worked alone.

Today they are ripping off black women in this country to the tune of $9 billion. The chemical **Products Manufacturers** are selling women of color destroys their hair. It dries out the hair so excessively that there is nothing that will reverse this dryness. Therefore, the inevitable consequence is that the hair pops and breaks. And, most black women will buy and use this No-Lye Relaxer Kit and "self-apply" the chemical by combing it through their hair. This method of application requires trying to straighten the same hair repeatedly. **Product Manufacturers** and many other white-owned companies sell her cheap oils, cheap shampoos, and cheap conditioners that don't stand a chance in hell of working. There is still much more...

The only way she can have hair is with a wig, a weave made of synthetic hair, braids, or by wearing a "boy" haircut. Now she must return to the same Korean stores where she buys more than 80 percent of this chemical that is not a relaxer. This time she buys volumes of cheap synthetic hair. Black women spend so much money collectively because they are desperately searching for ways to get their hair to grow. Yet, at the same time they are combing this chemical through their hair every four to eight weeks because the "new growth" must be relaxed, even with having a weave or braids.

This No-Lye Relaxer Kit has taken all of the business away from many thousands of black-owned Salons, and black manufacturers. These black salons were owned mostly by mothers of single parent households. The Beauty Giants have actually put them out of business and taken thousands of jobs away from black mothers who were trying to make a decent living for their families.

An Unknown Fact about Hair Conditioners and Shampoos

There are very few people who understand what **Conditioners** and **Shampoos** are for and how they work. Most Women will tell you that they buy whatever is the **cheapest Shampoo** and **Conditioner** on the market. If possible, they will try and find both the **Shampoo and Conditioner** in one container. This way they can shampoo the hair, rinse, and the work is done. If their hair starts to shed, break, and fall out, they will blame it on stress, being pregnant, or something they did or their Hairdresser did last week. But they will never admit that they have been using **cheap Shampoos** and **cheap Conditioners**! Most will buy a gallon for $5 to $8. And some will use it every day.

When There Is a Chemical No-Lye Relaxer in Black Hair none of the quality Hair Care Products on the following list will have any effect on a black woman's hair: Nexxus, Redken, American Crew, Nioxin, Mizani, Matrix, Redken, Alberto VO5, Beverly Johnson, Bumble & Bumble, Sebastian, L'Oreal, Revlon, John Frieda, Paul Mitchell, Pantene, Helen of Troy, Dudley's Q, or Goldwell Hair Care Products. Yet where there IS a **Chemical Lye Relaxer** found in the hair, all of the Hair Care Products on this list would be some of the best that money can buy and all would work exceptionally well!

Cheap hair products are totally worthless! Yet even if you use the **Very Best Hair Care Product** on the market, they will have absolutely NO effect on Black Hair after it has been chemically relaxed with a **Chemical No-Lye Relaxer Kit** because of the exceptionally, extreme DRYNESS it causes in the hair. **Cheap Black Hair Product** and Cheap White Product are about the same, and neither is worth a damn.

In other words, **Cheap Hair Product** will cause a black woman's hair to fall out quicker than she can say **"Cheap Black Hair Product!"** I recommend everything on the list above if there is not a No-Lye Relaxer in the hair. The products on the list will keep the hair as healthy as possible when used regularly every four to five days and more often where there is time in your busy schedule!

Chapter 13

ShamBOOsie's Texture Waving Technique

No Scalp Burns ever, guaranteed, and no guess-work:

The Texturizer is a technique *for use on Natural Hair, only.* With the retouch the chemical must be applied ONLY on your New Growth, and the best type of chemical to use is **Regular LYE Relaxer,** that is not sold in a kit. You need to purchase the **Regular LYE Relaxer** and a neutralizing shampoo in separate containers. A **No-Lye Relaxer Kit** will NOT work! It will ONLY destroy your hair! If your hair has been chemically relaxed already, it cannot be **Texturized.** If there is a No Relaxer Kit in your hair already, your hair cannot be **Texturized.** The technique must be used on *Natural Hair ONLY!*

A BURN Notice! First remember to never shampoo your hair before applying chemical relaxer, the scalp becomes very sensitive and will burn really bad, in all of five minutes. You must always allow about four days between shampooing and conditioning your hair, and getting the retouch relaxer or **ShamBOOsie's Texture Waving Application**. The hair will become clean by the end of the retouch process. When you give or receive a Texturizer, the idea is to NOT allow the hair to become straight! Oil, dirt, or gel on the hair will do more to help the process as long as the hair strands are loose and not stuck together.

It is very important **NOT** to use a **Box Kit or a No-Lye Relaxer Kit.** The **Conditioning Lye Relaxer** is much better. If you use a No-Lye Relaxer Kit, the chemical will have little or no effect on the hair because the No-Lye Relaxer destroys or neutralizes the natural bonds of the hair the first time around. Remember, a texturizer is simply a chemical relaxer, and when the chemical is left on the hair too long it will straighten the hair. With each retouch the chemical MUST be applied to the new growth only.

When the hair is *"NATURAL"* it will be necessary to gently pull a *WIDE-TOOTH COMB* through the hair, but only when there is not a chemical in the hair. Never Comb the Chemical through the hair during a Relaxer Retouch Texturizer; the chemical is applied to the New Growth ONLY and allowed to rest on the hair for about eight to ten minutes! NEVER Self-Apply your own Chemical and finally, NEVER use a Chemical NO-LYE Relaxer Kit!

ShamBOOsie's Texture Waving is very difficult to do over and over because each time the chemical is applied to hair that was previously treated with the chemical, that hair would relax a little more and maybe become straight. It takes a level of expertise to perform the process repeatedly. The Chemical must be applied to the New Growth ONLY, with each retouch, so you will need a little help from a friend. **It takes two baby—one to APPLY while one relaxes.**

If you have virgin hair, meaning NO Chemical LYE Relaxer is in your hair, your hair is natural. This is the only type of hair that can receive **ShamBOOsie's Texture Waving.** You are using a Chemical Relaxer so **ShamBOOsie's Texture Waving** does not CURL or put CURL in the hair; it REMOVES Curl. If the chemical is left on your hair longer than ten minutes, the chemical will straighten the hair. This is a better system for making your daughter's hair easier to manage, by removing about 70 percent of the natural CURL from the hair.

The chemical is applied to ALL the hair at once and then you gently use a wide-tooth comb to comb through the hair. When there is only WAVE left, which you will be able to see as you gently pull the comb through hair, rinse. After ten minutes, rinse no matter what. If there is any type of chemical, even a NO-Lye Relaxer Kit in the hair, **ShamBOOsie's Texture Waving** will NOT work. The hair must always be natural hair. Good luck.

A Chemical Tip:

Promise you will never put relaxer on your own hair because it is dangerous! The problem is that when you do your own retouch, you cannot see all of your New Growth well enough to apply the chemical ONLY on the New Growth. It is simply a lovely thing that you have New Growth, so why would anyone buy something that is supposed to make their hair Grow? It won't Grow! With the texturizer, the chemical has to be applied quickly and when it's time it has to be removed quickly. It is the first time the chemical should be applied with the fingers because it needs to be on the hair in one or two minutes. The retouch application is very different and works almost the same way as a regular retouch.

The chemical is applied ONLY to the new growth the same as with the retouch doing the regular application, but it too must be applied quickly. The person applying the product cannot do any talking while working because this will slow the process down. Sometimes, thirty seconds or one minute with the Chemical on the hair is too long because it can cause the hair to be relaxed straight, which cannot be reversed. When you do your own texturizer, you are forced to comb the chemical through the hair that has already been treated with the relaxer or the hair will end up straight during the process!

The art of chemically texturizing overly curly hair involves knowing a few secrets about the way the chemical works, its effect on the hair, and what actually takes place throughout the process. Combing during a Chemical Process doesn't add one thing to the process except it causes the hair to stretch and become very thin and smaller in diameter. All of the bonds in the hair that cause it to be overly curly will be altered and gone forever. This is why if the chemical is left on the hair too long it will straighten the hair, and the hair will not revert. It takes between twelve to fifteen minutes for hair to totally relax straight, starting from the time the chemical first comes in contact with the first section of the hair.

The process is "eyes on because it's a guessing game! You are looking for a soft wave or S shape curl in the hair. With the rinsing process, the chemical should be totally removed from the hair in about one minute. To take longer, may cause the hair to become straight. Remember, it's a guessing game and something could go wrong at any time. Everyone's hair will react differently depending the texture and strength of the hair.

This Is Very Important!

The entire scalp and a full inch around the hairline and the ears MUST be covered with an oil base, Vitamin AD&E from Dudley's Products! A tingling sensation could occur in the area of the first section where the application began. At any rate, look for the curl in the hair to start getting weaker in about 10 minutes after applying the Chemical.

A Chemical Tip:

Partial Relaxation in eight to ten minutes with "NO BURNS" guaranteed. The person applying the chemical must keep their eyes on the hair at all times. Never allow the hair to "go straight." Stand the wide-tooth comb straight up of its teeth and slowly pull the comb through the hair and watch the curl pattern in the hair.

There must be an S shape type of wave in the hair just before it's ready to be rinsed. A wide-tooth comb, not a fine-tooth comb, should be used. The wide-tooth comb will allow you to see the wave pattern. The process must be done with precision, and in a series of exact steps, in order to achieve the desired results. The same procedures for application and neutralization must be used every time the service is performed, without exception.

The Most Common Causes of Scalp Burns

1. Scratching the scalp with the finger nails a few days before having the hair relaxed. The itching that is often experienced is the scalp's way of telling you it's time for a retouch.
2. Shampooing the hair the day of or the day before the hair is to be relaxed. Make every effort not to touch the scalp or shampoo the hair the week before relaxer service is to be performed.
3. Not basing the scalp. Most people, including professionals, believe that when the package says "No Base" it means you should not base the scalp before applying this very hot chemical, a lye relaxer. The thing I do not understand is why it does not occur to them that this is a large part of the reason why the scalp is "set on fire" so quickly.
4. Leaving the chemical on the scalp too long. This is one of the greatest reasons of all. If 100 people perform this service, it will be performed 100 different ways, and chances are greater than 98 percent of them will leave the chemical on the scalp too long.

5. Having the service done just after sweating from exercising or swimming or doing anything to cause the scalp to become wet. Wetness of any kind will always cause the scalp to burn.

6. Combing the chemical through the hair irritates the scalp and will cause the scalp to burn.

7. Using the wrong strength and the wrong type of relaxer for your hair.

8. The home relaxer kit, the "kitchen perm." The kitchen is NOT the best place to do this service because the facilities are not adequate and there are some imminent safety hazards. If you must relax the hair at home, buy all of your products separately not in a kit. Read all of the directions before starting **ShamBOOsie's Texture Waving Technique. Use a Regular LYE Relaxer – Not a Kit, it will destroy your hair!**

9. This is the greatest reason of all. The person performing the service, including professional stylists, does not know how to use the chemical relaxer properly. Application with most of them is "a guessing game" so be very careful!

A ShamBOOsie Chemical Tip: ALWAYS base the entire scalp every time before **ShamBOOsie's Texture Wave** and use a base that is designed for that purpose. The Chemical to use for **ShamBOOsie's Texture Waving** is a Conditioning LYE Relaxer. Most LYE Relaxers will do the JOB just fine. The "LYE" Relaxer is also referred to as "Sodium Hydroxide," which should be written on the label. You will also need a neutralizing shampoo and Vitamin AD&E to base the scalp.

Rinse very well after each application of the shampoo, use a generous amount of the Neutralizing Shampoo, make the lather as thick as possible and leave the last one on the hair for a full ten minutes, set a timer, rinse, and condition the hair. To wear **ShamBOOsie's**

Texture Wave, buy Pink Oil and use sparingly. You may also use a large fine-tooth comb, with a Blow Dryer or a Blow Dryer with a comb attachment to run through damp hair. Apply some Crème Press Hairdressing, lightly to every strand of your hair, spray on some medium hold spray styling, section the hair and use a ceramic flat iron. It's MAGIC!

Be sure you completely understand the application method before you begin an application of a Chemical Hair Relaxer, including the application of a Texturizer. This is the proper way to chemically relax hair with absolutely No Breakage, No Overprocessing, No Combing, and No Scalp Burns.

A Chemical Tip: Timing Is the Key.

Timing is the most important element in this service. Do not take this lightly. Be aware of your working time during the entire application process. **Use a timer please!**

Remember:

The timing begins with the start of the first application the moment relaxer touches the hair and ends with the beginning of the first rinse.

A Chemical Tip: Towel blot all excess water from the rinsing process, and change the towel around the neck before neutralizing, to prevent breakage in the nape area due to residual chemical left in the towel.

A Chemical Tip: Proper neutralization and conditioning are essential for any finished look. They should be done the proper way every time.

A Chemical Tip: You must Completely Stop the Action of the Chemical to avoid losing the hair. Failure to completely stop the action of the chemical will leave the chemical working for hours after the hair has been styled and finished, and loss of hair will be inevitable. You must towel blot all excess water from the hair after each rinse, so as to not dilute the Neutralizer. The neutralizing shampoo is *a neutralizer in shampoo form*, and it does not wash the chemical from the hair.

When applying the neutralizing shampoo, use a generous amount. (The lather should feel like whipped cream). Do three shampoo applications, massage well, pay special attention to the nape area, and leave the last neutralizing shampoo in the hair for five minutes. Set a timer.

Apply a conditioner and leave in for a full five minutes. If a dryer is needed, cover the head with a plastic cap and place under a "warm dryer" for ten to fifteen minutes.

A Chemical Tip: Hot stuff!

If you shampoo the hair first and then realize that you were supposed to do a relaxer, do not dry the hair and attempt to apply the relaxer! Doing so will certainly cause severe scalp burns in the first five minutes. The same will occur if the person receiving the relaxer gets caught in the rain, went swimming or did a shampoo earlier the same day of the relaxer or even the day before.

Chapter 14

A Healthier, Safer, and More Comfortable Way to Relax Hair

A Hair Wellness Approach to Relaxing Hair guarantees NO Scalp Burns Ever! No Hair Damage or Extreme Dryness of the Hair and No Guesswork. It's an accurate, painless, step-by-step application process. There are reasons why I have such a detailed knowledge of hair. I remember all the mistakes I have made over the years, and I remember all the successes I have had over the years. I have tried hundreds of different types of oils, shampoos, gels, hair sprays, and CONDITIONERS, so I know what works and what does not work. I never do anything to hair without knowing exactly what and why I am doing it.

Your Hair Should Be Relaxed Only Once in Its Lifetime

This may sound impossible because NEW hair is continuously GROWING, so allow me to explain! The new growth is the ONLY HAIR that should need to be Chemically Relaxed. If you do the job correctly every time, you should not have to reapply relaxer. *Your hair should be relaxed only once in its lifetime, no matter how long your hair GROWS and this is the healthiest way to manage the process.* How many times do you think you can straighten or relax the same hair over and over again before it all falls out? Everyone, including many Hairdressers, is doing it the wrong way by combing the Chemical through the hair over and over again.

This application method and every concept mentioned is the EXACT process that I perform on clients in the salon. The collection of light OILS, Crèmes, Conditioners, Shampoos, Gels, Hair Styling Sprays, and tools are recommended in all of my hair care Books. **ShamBOOsie's Hair Wellness Approach to Hair Growth** will fulfill every need and every concept because the methodology has been tested a thousand times.

I fully understand every product that I use; I know its chemistry and its positive and negative effects on your hair. I never guess about any of it. What I don't know, I will research and study until I have perfected that area of knowledge. To learn to cut hair I had to cut a thousand different haircuts, some of them ten times, to get them perfect. (The chemical relaxer must be applied, removed and neutralized with absolute perfection every time!)

ShamBOOsie Notices Things Usually Overlooked by Most!

I am dyslexic, which allows me to see HAIR in three dimensions. I see and teach everything about HAIR in minute detail, and I will point out things that are usually overlooked by most people. I view this as a gift from God that helps me have a greater understanding of how your hair really works—how to protect it and how to CARE for it. You can't argue with Science and Chemistry, and it makes no sense to play a guessing game with Chemicals, Conditioners, and cheap hair products. If you do, you will lose your hair. This entire Book is about helping you GROW and have the most healthy, most beautiful HAIR of your lifetime.

You Must First Build a Conditioning LYE Relaxer Kit from Scratch!

I am constantly asked where to find a *Conditioning LYE Relaxer KIT*. There is no such kit on the market, so the person applying the Chemical must put one together. It is very simple to build one and every component must be purchased separately. You will need:

- A sixteen-ounce jar of chemical relaxer: Lye (Regular Strength)
- A bottle of neutralizing shampoo
- Oil base – **ShamBOOsie** uses Vitamin AD&E from Dudley's Products
- Six salon towels
- A shampoo cape
- Rubber gloves
- Two rat-tail combs
- Two plastic caps

The **NO-LYE Relaxer Kit** is **NOT** a part of this or of any part of what this book teaches. If you intend to use a **NO-LYE Relaxer Kit** throw this book in the garbage! The **NO-LYE Relaxer Kit** does one thing, it destroys your hair!

You must promise to **NEVER Self-Apply and NEVER Comb** another **Chemical No-Lye Relaxer** Kit or any other type of Chemical through your own hair or you will continue to lose your hair! The problem most black women have with the Chemical Relaxer is they don't know how the Chemical Relaxer works or that combing the Chemical through their hair does damage that cannot be reversed. Just about everyone selects the wrong types of Chemicals for the work that needs to be done.

First and foremost: **"The Black Woman and her Daughters must Master the Art of Applying the Chemical LYE Relaxer, which guarantees No Scalp Burns Ever!"**

A Conditioning LYE Relaxer is the best and safest chemical to use. Otherwise it's like taking someone else's medication and not knowing how it will affect you. Just as the wrong medicine can kill you, using the wrong types of chemicals the wrong way can "kill your hair."

You do not save money by using NO-Lye Relaxer Kits and **Self-Applying Chemical Relaxer.** You actually increase the cost of caring for your hair ten fold by buying cheap hair products to try and undo the damage! The Chemical Manufacturers love having you use a **NO-LYE Relaxer Kit** because they know it will damage your hair and that you will buy everything in sight to try and stop the loss of your hair! They have designed the Chemicals just for this purpose; to make you spend money on maintenance hair products that they know are cheap and will never deliver. This book is written to change all that and set you on the right path for success.

Most LYE Relaxers will probably contain built-in conditioners. I coined the phrase, **"Conditioning Lye Relaxer"** to indicate that it is milder and that it is the best chemical for your hair. When purchasing, simply ask for a *LYE* Relaxer. On the back of the label will be the words, **Sodium Hydroxide!** Some Lye Relaxers will come with a thick liquid called a Normalizer and a Neutralizing Shampoo, which is a Neutralizer in shampoo form.

The thick liquid Normalizer is always applied first to bring the pH of the hair down as close to seven on the pH scale as possible. This will prevent the hair from becoming dry. (Not the kind of dryness found in **No Lye** Relaxer.) Follow the directions on the container.

Next the Neutralizer in shampoo form must be handled an EXACT way to be effective. Remember, this is the product that will completely STOP the Lye Relaxer from working, so you want the Neutralizing Shampoo to work very well. You want the chemical to STOP working. Use the Neutralizer Shampoo EXACTLY as this book teaches. No exceptions!

Stop Relaxing Your Own Hair at Home!

The first change to make is to stop **combing** relaxer through your own hair. This process will destroy your hair and cause you to lose ALL your hair. Although this book illustrates the proper application technique for applying chemical relaxer, I DO NOT recommend you do the relaxer service at home and certainly not on your own hair. Chemical services such as applying Permanent hair color, Relaxers, and Curls should be done by a Salon Professional.

A ShamBOOsie Chemical TIP!

If you can get this process of managing your hair right EVERY TIME, there is no reason why you shouldn't be able to GROW longer, healthier, more beautiful hair and keep it that way. The secret is in the application process. Every item of concern throughout the step-by-step application process must be followed to the letter without exception!

Combing the Chemical through the Hair Is Dangerous!

- The chemical MUST be the right strength and the right type—**LYE**!
- The base oil you MUST put on the scalp MUST be the right type—**Vitamin AD&E**!
- The step-by-step Application Process MUST be followed to the letter.

- The "TIMING" process MUST be Precise, with no exceptions! This means the chemical MUST be applied and rinsed in a timely fashion—applied to the hair in ten minutes, (two and one-half minutes per section); rinsed ACCURATELY and in a TIMELY fashion to ensure the straightening of the hair is processed without error.
- The neutralizing process is more important than the application process. If you err, you will lose all of the hair.
- READ every word of the instructions below, three to four times before you start and keep the step-by-step application instructions in your face throughout the process.
- Every step of this application process must be without error—no exceptions!

ShamBOOsie's Step-by-Step Relaxer Application Method Follow My Directions to the Letter...

AGAIN! The person applying the relaxer MUST read *all* the instructions below before starting the relaxer application. The very second any chemical comes in contact with the hair, is when the chemical starts to work, no matter where the chemical touches the hair. YOU must control the entire process. **This chemical is nothing to play with; it will take out all of your hair if handled incorrectly.**

1. Section the hair into four sections, parting the hair down the center of the head, from front to back and from ear to ear. Twist and clip each of the four sections into place.
2. **BASING THE SCALP!** This is one of the most important phases of the process and it MUST be done extremely well. Every inch of the scalp MUST be covered with the basing oil. **ShamBOOsie** uses Vitamin AD&E from Dudley's Products.
3. **NEVER** apply chemical around the face and hairline FIRST. This will cause balding temples! You want to cover the entire scalp, a full inch beyond the hairline and be sure to also cover the ears.

4. Start the application at the back of the head. Remember to **NEVER** apply the chemical around **ALL** the partings separating the sections; instead work with a single section at a time. Complete the first section then move to the next! You cannot control the timing or the way the chemical works by doing it any other way.

5. Not having complete control of the chemical while it's on the hair and scalp, will cause scalp burns everywhere the chemical is on the hair and scalp. Again, the chemical starts working the moment it touches the hair and scalp. The proper way is to apply chemical to each section separately as you progress.

6. Each time you finish applying chemical to one section, move on to the next section. Stay in control.

7. Starting the application: apply the chemical completely around the first section in the BACK on the left side on the head. Outline ONLY this section. Next do the first horizontal partings, starting at the TOP and *using the back of the comb,* apply chemical on the UPPER portion of the parting ONLY and be generous with the product! The idea is to get the first application on the hair in just ten minutes.

Now make the second horizontal parting, and apply chemical on the UPPER portion of the parting ONLY, then do the same thing until you complete the first quarter section. There is no need to apply chemical on the lower half of the parting because it will be covered each time you apply chemical to the next parting. Move on to the quarter section on the back RIGHT side of the back of the head and repeat the application process of the first quarter section.

Using the back of the comb! Apply the chemical completely around the second quarter section in the BACK of the head on the RIGHT side. Outline ONLY this quarter section. Next do the first horizontal partings, starting at the TOP and apply chemical on the UPPER portion of the parting ONLY, be generous with the product!

Do a second horizontal parting, and apply chemical on the UPPER portion ONLY, then do the same thing until you complete the second quarter section. Again, there is no need to apply chemical on the lower half of the parting because it will be covered each time you apply chemical to the next parting. Move on to the quarter section on the Front RIGHT side of the head and repeat the application process of the first quarter section in the back, with one exception.

Using the back of the comb! This time apply the chemical completely around the third quarter section on the front of the head on the RIGHT side, BUT DONNOT apply chemical on the face and hairline, do it LAST on the Front RIGHT side of the head as you are applying chemical on the horizontal partings. This way you avoid leaving chemical on the face too long and avoid burns around the face. Cover just the third section and then move on to the fourth and final section, remember to NOT apply chemical on the face and hairline, do it LAST on the Front LEFT side of the head. The reason, the facial skin is extremely sensitive, and of a different type that the skin on the scalp. Read this section again until it's understood...

A ShamBOOsie Chemical Tip!

Do not smooth those vertical partings between the quarter-sections, but use the back of the comb, and smooth ONLY the horizontal partings! If you should go through and smooth the vertical partings anyway, those partings will show up in the comb out and finished look. It will take you a week to get them out of the hair!

Why Is Smoothing Necessary?

The only way to check and determine if the Chemical Relaxer is doing its JOB is to use a technique I call "Smoothing." **No Combing EVER!** Use the back of the comb to Smooth where the Chemical is between the horizontal partings, **New Growth** just as you did while applying the Chemical during the first application. Smoothing ONLY the horizontal partings also allows you to see where you need to add or apply more Chemical Relaxer on the "New Growth ONLY" you will miss a few spots the time around. Please remember to be generous with the Chemical Relaxer Crème, to make sure there is enough to get the job done. **Allow the Chemical to DO ALL THE WORK!**

NEVER Smooth between the vertical parting—NEVER! They are only there to give you more control of the process. Smoothing between the vertical partings will cause the finished look to have unwanted separations that will take a week to remove.

No Combing EVER! The reason for "Smoothing" is NOT to help the Chemical Relaxer do its job; the relaxer is capable of doing ALL of its own work. However, smoothing allows you to see that the hair being relaxed is becoming smooth and silky, as it lies next to the scalp. If the hair has NOT relaxed properly, as you smooth with the back of the comb, look closely and you will notice the hair will lift slightly each time you smooth the New Growth, telling you that the Chemical Relaxer needs to remain on the hair longer. The first Application should take about two minutes to two and one-half minutes per section to complete, and about ten minutes to cover the entire head. If it takes two minutes, that's okay; COUNT it as ten minutes anyway. Some women will have thinner or less hair, and some will have much more.

The Process Is Time-Sensitive So Set a Timer!
For the first Application!

1. The fourth section in the front of the head, the Chemical Relaxer has been on the hair for about **two and one-half minutes.**

2. The third section in the front of the head, the Chemical Relaxer has been on the hair for about **five minutes.**

3. The second section in the back of the head, the Chemical Relaxer has been on the hair for about **seven and one-half minutes.**

4. The first section in the back of the head, the Chemical Relaxer has been on the hair for about **ten minutes.**

The Chemical Relaxer has been on her hair for about ten minutes in the first section in back of the head. This section is the time element you will use to determine the amount of time before starting the rinsing process of the Chemical Relaxer.

The second application is to check for missing areas; it will go faster, about one to one and one-half minutes per section! Be generous with the Chemical Relaxer; you have about six minutes to finish and when added to the first ten minutes, it means the chemical Relaxer has been on the first section of the hair for about sixteen minutes total.

You want to go through the hair smoothing a third time, by now she should start to feel a slight tingling in the first section ONLY. It is now getting very close to the time for removing or rinsing the Chemical Relaxer. If at any time she feels tingling or burning anywhere else on her head, it is because she was scratching her scalp before, or the scalp was not based very well, or this could just be a sensitive area.

NEVER ask, "Is it burning?" If you do, she will start to burn all over her head. Even a slight tingling will be interpreted as burning. Instead ask, **"Are you all right?"** or **"Are you comfortable?"** Remember, she is expecting to burn because she always has with everyone else, but this is a **No Burn EVER Application Process!**

1. When *Smoothing—NOT combing* make horizontal partings as with the first application. *using the back of the comb!* Go through each section using horizontal partings and using to BACK of the comb. Be sure to apply more chemical where it's needed to make sure all the New GROWTH is covered with chemical.

   You are smoothing to see how fast the chemical is working, not to get the hair straighter. The relaxer will do all the work of relaxing your hair. Smoothing the vertical partings between the sections will cause the hair to separate down the middle of the head and from ear to ear in the finished look. In other words, it will mess up the style, and it could take a week or two to get rid of those separations in the hair.

2. Start by applying chemical to the outline of the first section in the back of the head first. Start on the left or right side, but do it this way every time so as to form a memory of the application system. (Remember, each section of the hair is handled separately. This means the chemical should not be applied to any other areas of the head).

3. Next, at the top of the first section make one-quarter-inch horizontal partings and apply the chemical to the top half of each parting ONLY. (Use a liberal amount of the chemical to get the job done. This will add speed to the application process.)

4. The bottom side of the part will share the chemical of the top half when the next part is made and chemical is applied to the top half of that parting.

5. Handle each section exactly the same way, with one exception. When applying chemical to outline the two front sections, it is

very important to leave the area around the hairline and face for last in each section as you go. (You want the product on the face as short a time as possible.)

6. The chemical should be applied to this area at the completion of each separate section in the front as you go. In other words, this area should be last, after all of the other hair has been covered, at end of the third section, and then at the end of the fourth section.

7. The skin around the hairline and face is more sensitive to the chemical. This is where the scalp and facial skin meet. Facial skin is softer with many more sweat and oil glands, so burns will occur much quicker in this area. The hair around the face is drier and more resistant as a result of washing the face every day. The hair is more fragile with a texture much like baby hair.

8. NEVER COMB chemical through the hair around the face. You will go bald in this area if you do. This hair will be the first to go when the shedding and breakage begins.

The Rinsing Process is Time-Sensitive Set a Timer!

The rinsing process starts with the first section, where the application process began. Since the relaxer wasn't applied to all of the hair at the same time, it must NOT be removed ALL AT ONCE, it must be removed in the same order it was applied.

Rinse the first section in the back of the head, a FULL two minutes before moving on to the second section. (Set a timer!) A FULL two minutes gives the second and third sections time for the Chemical Relaxer to complete its work, relaxing the hair. This way when it's all said and done ALL of the hair, all of the New Growth on entire head of hair will have had time to be completely relaxed. So, rinse the first section of the hair for a FULL two minutes or maybe two and one-half minutes if needed, to ensure the hair is relaxed. Keep your eyes on the work to determine if the next section is ready to be rinsed.

If for some reason she starts to really burn, remove ALL the Chemical, if necessary, to keep her from burning or remove just the spot where she is burning. This is another reason why using a Conditioning LYE Relaxer is so much better, you can always go back and complete the job the next time around. **This is NOT possible to do with a No-Lye Relaxer Kit!** It may be possible to remove the chemical ONLY from the area where she is burning.

Move on to the second section and rinse for two FULL minutes, and then move on to the third section and rinse for a FULL two minutes, BUT remove the Chemical from around the face.

The entire process should take between twenty-two and twenty-four minutes, with NO SCALP BURNS EVER!

Important Rules to Remember

- The chemical relaxer starts to work the very moment it comes in contact with the hair, scalp, and facial skin.
- The idea is to properly and completely straighten *all* the hair without scalp burns, without overprocessing (damaging the hair) or underprocessing any portion of the hair.
- The first application, all the way through all the hair, must be completed in ten minutes, about two and one-half minutes per section.
- The person applying the chemical should set a timer for ten minutes and work without talking because concentration must be focused on the application and the time element.

A Chemical Tip:
- **Never COMB** the chemical through the hair for any reason. Do not comb the hair while chemical is on the hair for any reason

or you will cause the hair to become thin, weak and break. But don't take my word for it, just take a look in the mirror at your hair and see for yourself! The chemical is designed to do ALL of its own work. Just apply the chemical to the "New GROWTH ONLY!"

- Be gentle with the hair, but work with speed, keeping the chemical under control and in the area of the *new growth only,* as much as possible. Do not skimp on the product, use as much as you need so that the chemical can work.
- You will miss some spots along the way but you can catch them the second time around.
- Apply more chemical as needed and cover every tiny piece of hair around the hairline and the back of the head (the nape area).

A ShamBOOsie Warning

Remember that the hair is very fragile while it is being chemically relaxed, and combing stretches the hair, which cannot be seen with the naked eye, but will cause breakage. So *never* comb the chemical through the hair. *The hair is being chemically straightened, not straightened by any physical means.* So no combing is necessary. The chemical is designed to do all of its own work. All you need to do is apply it properly.

- The second application through the hair is to make sure that *all* the hair is covered. The second application will go much faster, and take only about five minutes to complete the entire head.
- Again, using fresh HORIZONTAL partings start with the first section in the back of the head, working from the top down.
- Make thin HORIZONTAL subsections, and apply additional chemical where needed to the TOP SIDE of the HORIZONTAL partings only, for faster application.

- The smoothing is done as the relaxer is applied. Remember, timing is the key.
- The third time through is smoothing only. It will take about two minutes to complete.
- The subject may feel a bit of "tingling" at this point, where the chemical was first applied. This is your signal that the hair is about ready to be rinsed and that the possibility of scalp burns is eminent.
- Remember, each application should be applied all the way *to the scalp* but *not on the scalp*. This will take practice but will become easier over time. Don't talk; just apply.
- During a new growth retouch application, the hair to be relaxed is **only the new growth**, which is the hair closest to the scalp. The rest of the hair is already straight. The chemical will move a little, but do not comb it through to the ends of the hair. The chemical cannot break down the bonds again where the bonds have already been destroyed or broken down.
- In basic Cosmetology schools students are taught to apply the chemical one-quarter inch off the scalp. This is **not** the proper way because the hair being relaxed *is* that one-quarter inch of new growth. That one-quarter inch of hair requires the entire thirteen to fifteen minutes of processing time to be relaxed properly.

A Healthier, Safer and More Comfortable Way to Relax Hair is the solution to the problems you have been having with chemical relaxers. Learn the application method, and it will work for you every time, with NO scalp burns EVER! After following this application method a few times, the steps will come naturally and become easier. Share this information with friends and family. Remember, **"It takes two baby—me and you, It takes two!"**

More Important Things to Remember

- Always examine the scalp for scratches and abrasions **before** applying any chemical to the hair and scalp.
- Always section the hair into four equal sections. The sections that are not being worked on should be clipped up and out of the way.
- Always apply protective base to the *entire* scalp and one inch around the face, hairline, ears, and nape area, leaving no dry spots. Check the scalp before you start.
- Use only Vitamin AD&E Hair & Scalp Oil by Dudley Products for basing the scalp. This product was designed specifically for this purpose as well as many other uses. Petroleum jelly or hair grease should never be used because they are too heavy and may interfere with the chemical process.
- Always wear protective gloves at all times or your fingers will swell, turn purple, and hurt badly. There will be nothing you can do to stop the pain. (I know because I have broken this rule.)

When the hair is properly relaxed, it will lay down on the scalp. If the hair is not properly relaxed, it will rise up slightly off the scalp as you smooth. When the hair is relaxed, it will feel silky and very soft to the touch. If it feels hard to the touch when it's time to remove the chemical, give it one or two more minutes. If the hair is not relaxed by the end of the two minutes, start the rinsing process anyway. If the hair is not properly relaxed, it will revert to curly or wavy after the first shampoo and conditioner a week later.

A ShamBOOsie Awareness TIP! When you are relaxing hair that has previously been relaxed with *No-Lye Relaxer* and the hair was not properly straightened, the No-Lye Relaxer will "lock in" the remaining curl pattern in the hair. When this happens, nothing, no other chemical or anything will be able to break this hair down and remove the curl. The reason is because the bonds were destroyed without getting the hair straight. The only hair that will become straight is the new GROWTH hair closest to the scalp.

Technically Speaking
The No-Lye Relaxer is a Very Dangerous Chemical

Take a look around you. It seems as if most women of color and even little Black Girls everywhere, are wearing **False Hair.** These hair extensions are attached to the very short hair that is left after the use and misuse of the **No-Lye Relaxer** and other chemicals. **No-Lye Relaxer** chemically locks the cuticle layer of the hair, preventing anything else from entering the cortex layer, thus altering its texture. Most conditioners and oil moisturizers, no matter how well they are made, will have little or no effect on the dryness caused by the **No-Lye Relaxer.**

Research has determined that women of color collectively spend **$9 billion** yearly trying to find a way to relaxing their hair, relieve the dryness, and keep the hair healthy, and GROWING.

The only solution some women have put their trust in up to this point has been OIL, and lots of it! Addressing this problem requires very special products—an assortment of moisturizing conditioning formulas. Few product companies, however, have sought to make a line of products that work. The stronger and coarser the hair, the drier, harder, and more brittle the hair will become after using the **No-Lye Relaxer!**

THE ONLY THING THAT WILL WORK is what I call the Magic Formula, which is my method of application and selection of just the right kind and PERFECT products. Then simply follow my lead. This is a mixture of Shampoos, a short list of very high quality

Beautiful Black Hair

Conditioners, and a light oil moisturizing hairdressing. The **No-Lye Relaxer** is a silent man-made hair "disease" and "destroyer." There is a common misunderstanding that the **No-Lye Relaxer** is "better" for the hair than the Conditioning Lye Relaxer—that is "the real lie." Extreme dryness from No-Lye Relaxer is irreversible in most cases and next to impossible to control. With the right moisturizing conditioners, the right kind of hairdressing, and a few other specially formulated maintenance products, the dryness can be controlled. Over time, with the proper care, the damaged hair *can* be replaced with newly grown healthier hair.

The Virgin Relaxer Retouch and a Corrective Application

They are applied the same way. The process of applying a Conditioning Lye Relaxer over a **No-Lye Relaxer**, (which I recommend) is called a **Corrective Retouch**. The hair must be prepared, treated, strengthened, and conditioned very well before doing this service. The same must take place before every retouch from this moment forward. You can expect minimal shedding but don't be alarmed. For the corrective relaxer and the virgin relaxer, the chemical must be applied to the entire length of the hair shaft. Remember, timing is the key and it remains the same with the application of every relaxer.

- When it is a **corrective relaxer**, you begin and complete the process the same as any retouch.
- After smoothing the third time, apply the chemical by hand to the rest of the hair and smooth with your fingers for only three to five minutes. (Be sure to wear gloves.)
- Then begin the rinsing process. The directions are to follow. The objective is to simply condition the hair that was previously relaxed with the No-Lye Relaxer, not to straighten the hair.

- However, if there is *Lye Relaxer* in all the hair, but the hair did not become relaxed in previous attempts, resort to the same process as with the *Corrective Retouch*. **Apply the chemical to all the hair that needs relaxing.** This may not be the full length of the hair.
- With a Virgin relaxer, use the same process as with a Retouch, except the chemical is applied to the *entire length* of the hair, one section at a time. You must get the product on the hair quickly. The smoothing is done with your fingers until the service is completed.
- Completing the service should take eighteen to twenty minutes when using a *mild*, twenty-two to twenty-four minutes with *regular*, and twenty-two minutes when using a *super* relaxer. The super should ONLY be applied to RESISTANT hair. **I have only used a super strength of chemical two or three times in my entire career.**
- **Keeping an Eye on Your Timing is a Must!**
- The timing begins with the start of the first application, which is the moment the chemical comes in contact with the first section of hair, and the time ends with the beginning of the rinse of the first section.
- Do not alter this method of rinsing; it is the key to getting all the hair straight, with NO BURNS ever.

A ShamBOOsie Chemical TIP: It is very important to use a *mild* relaxer every time when the hair has been permanently colored. No exceptions!

Relaxing Color-Treated Hair

Again, the hair MUST be prepared, treated, strengthened, and conditioned very well before doing this service. **The color-treated hair must be protected,** even if the new growth is not completely relaxed as straight as you would like. Be sure to coat the color-treated hair with Vitamin AD&E Hair and Scalp Oil. **This is the only instance**

when I will tell you to put oil on the hair. The oil will help to protect the hair before applying the relaxer, assuring that the chemical is kept in the area of the new growth. All of this is an absolute must!

An Imperative Chemical Tip!

Apply the chemical thoroughly on the new GROWTH and simply let the product sit on the hair. DO NOT SMOOTH with the back of the comb.

Another Imperative Chemical Tip!

A Warning: Even if you were using a *super* or a *regular* relaxer before having your hair permanently colored, use only a *mild* relaxer from this point on or until you GROW completely out of the color. (We are talking months!)

The Rinsing Process: Set a Timer

READ this section then READ it again! DO NOT CHANGE A THING.

When most of the hair has been sufficiently straightened, the rinse must be initiated in the same order as the application of the chemical.

- Starting with the first section, rinse only this section thoroughly for two full minutes before moving on to rinse the next section. Then rinse the second section for two full minutes. (Set a timer for ten minutes and keep an eye on the clock.)
- After the second section is completed, rinse both sections again for one full minute, before moving on to the third section. (This is a total of five full minutes).
- Rinse the third section for two full minutes. Then rinse all three sections for one full minute. (The total time is now eight minutes). Then proceed to the fourth section, and rinse this section with all the rest of the hair for two full minutes.

An Essential Chemical Tip!

Rinsing the hair in this manner will allow sections two, three, and four to have sufficient time to completely relax before the chemical is removed. The entire chemical was not applied at the same time, so you cannot begin the rinse anywhere you wish. The hair will not be completely relaxed at the same time, which means all the hair should not be rinsed at the same time and you must start where you began. This rinsing procedure is also the only way to ensure that *all* of the hair will be completely and properly processed.

Important Points to Keep in Mind

- Towel blot as much water as possible, and change the towel around the neck before the neutralizing process of the chemical begins. This will prevent breakage in the nape area because of residual chemical left in the soiled towel.
- Proper neutralization and proper conditioning are essential for any finished look. The neutralization process must completely stop the action of the chemical or it will eat right through your hair. It is the most important part of the process. The neutralization process must be followed exactly each time, no exceptions, no short cuts and no compromises.
- The chemical continues to work until you stop it or until it stops on its own, about six hours later. YOU MUST STOP THE ACTION! If the action of the chemical is not stopped, the loss of hair is inevitable.
- Towel blot all excess water from the hair after each rinse, after each neutralizer shampoo application, and do three applications of the neutralizing shampoo. Any water left on the hair after each rinse will dilute the neutralizing shampoo. You don't want anything to weaken this product. Full strength is so much better.

- When applying the neutralizing shampoo, use a generous amount. The lather must be the consistency of whipped cream all three times.
- Massage the scalp and the hair very well, paying special attention to the nape area. Then rinse very well, blot the excess water with a towel, and leave the third and final neutralizer on the hair for five full minutes. Set a timer!

A ShamBOOsie Chemical TIP!

The neutralizing shampoo is for *stopping the action of the chemical*. It is not a shampoo, but a *neutralizer in shampoo form* so that the neutralizer can be worked into a foam that will sit on the hair for a full five minutes.

Use a towel to blot the excess water after rinsing and apply a conditioner. Do not overdo it with the conditioner, use as much as you need, but don't waste it. Leave the conditioner in the hair for a full fifteen minutes. If the hair was previously relaxed with No-Lye Relaxer, and no hair color is involved, condition the hair with Humectress Moisturizing Conditioner. Cover the hair with a plastic cap, and sit under a warm dryer for fifteen minutes. Then rinse well, dry the hair, apply Crème Press Hairdressing, and style as usual.

More Important Points to Keep in Mind

- During the application, never *comb* the hair in an effort to aid the straightening process.
- When smoothing, always use a very light touch, and try not to move the chemical around more than necessary.
- Remember, it is the chemical breaking down of the bonds that relaxes and straightens the hair, not combing the chemical through the hair. Let the chemical do its JOB!

- If hair breakage is noticeable while smoothing, rinse the chemical out of the hair immediately. Do a conditioner treatment with a High-End concentrated moisturizing or protein conditioner followed by a quality moisturizing conditioner designed for damaged hair.
- Use Keraphix Protein Conditioner and Humectress Moisturizing Conditioner from Nexxus Products.
- Remember, the person receiving the chemical service should never be left unattended with the chemical on the hair or at any time during the chemical process.
- If any discomfort is felt, remove the chemical, even if the hair is not completely straightened. A sting, tingling, or an itch here or there is *not* the same as "burning."
- If there is a chemical reaction in just a small spot somewhere on the scalp, i.e., a sting, tingling, or an itch, use a wet towel to remove the chemical from that spot only, and spray some hairspray on the spot. The hairspray will cool the area for one to two minutes. It will also give you about two minutes, maybe, the time you need to finish the work. Continue to smooth and check the hair.
- Remember, if the hair is not in healthy condition, a series of conditioning treatments should be done three to four times for about two weeks, to make the hair stronger and to bring the hair back to a more tolerant state before the chemical relaxer. The hair must be able to sustain the application of the chemical.

Shampoo Before Relaxing and "Burn, Baby, Burn!"

If you have shampooed the hair the day of a retouch or the day before, do not do the retouch. If you do, the chemical will "Set your scalp on fire." If your hairdresser makes the mistake of wetting your hair, she should not attempt to dry the hair and apply the relaxer. Severe burning of the scalp is certain to occur in the first five to ten minutes. Once this happens you will not be able to remove the chemical quickly enough. The intensity of the burning will increase rapidly. The same will occur if you get caught in the rain, go swimming the same day, or the night before a retouch relaxer.

Don't Ever Forget This!

- Fine hair, damaged, and color-treated hair MUST be relaxed only with a *mild* relaxer. Be sure to apply the chemical to the New Growth ONLY.
- During a first-time or virgin relaxer (When the hair has never been relaxed before) the relaxer is applied to the entire length of the hair, all the way *to* the scalp but not *on* the scalp.
- Every type of chemical relaxer, Sodium Hydroxide, Thio, or Japanese, rearranges or completely changes the basic structure of the hair by breaking or destroying the disulfide bonds of the hair. The Japanese relaxer is not safe for use on black hair; it will cause the hair to break. The disulfide bonds that are destroyed or broken by Sodium Hydroxide relaxer can never be reformed. The hair is forever chemically straightened or altered.
- To neutralize the action of a Sodium Hydroxide relaxer, an acid-balanced shampoo is required. It is a NEUTRALIZER in shampoo form, *not* a shampoo for cleaning the hair!
- Never shampoo the hair before the application of a Sodium Hydroxide relaxer or within working days before service.
- The relaxer should be applied first to the hair in back of the head because the hair is normally more resistant in the back. Never apply relaxer around the face and hairline first! The skin is more sensitive in these areas.

Now, Relax and Enjoy the GROWTH of Your Hair.

Chapter 15

For Your Information

When there is Not a No-LYE Relaxer In Your Hair

Let's consider what is necessary to bring a single line of High Quality Hair CARE Products to market such as Dudley's **Quality Hair Care Products**, which is the best black-owned company in the business. Then there is Nexxus**, Paul Mitchell, John Frieda, Matrix**, Redken, Revlon, **and Hair Care Products.** When the hair is natural or when there is a **Chemical LYE Relaxer** in the hair all of the Quality Hair Care Products above will work very well to keep your hair in good condition. It is the fact that your relaxer is a LYE Relaxer that allows the hair to benefit from using these and other quality Conditioners and Shampoos. Notice that these are what you will call **"white hair care products."**

The moment you Comb a **NO-LYE Relaxer Kit** through your hair, all bets are off! PLEASE understand that Hair Products are about HAIR, **"As you are able to see it, with both eyes closed!"** The ones mentioned here are some of the best products in world, but not necessarily the best products for your hair because these products were not created with your extreme problems in mind. If you were "NOT" using a "No-Lye Relaxer" as your Chemical Hair Restructuring products, all of the wonderful Hair CARE Products mentioned above would be the perfect **Hair CARE** Products for your hair. Referring

Beautiful Black Hair

ONLY to the Conditioners and Shampoos! Your personal Hair CARE regimen is about the "Scientific Study" of the art of personal beautification. In other words, the product matches the needs of the hair...

This is one Ponzi scheme that affects every black woman in America. The Giant Hair Product Manufacturers will continue to sell you **Chemicals NO-LYE Relaxer Kits** that they know will both DRY your hair OUT and TAKE your hair OUT! Then they will sell you inferior quality conditioners that are useless, and tons of OILS that are useless, as a defense against the DRYNESS this chemical relaxer causes. No Giant Hair Product Manufacturers or any of the little companies MAKE a conditioner and shampoo that will save your hair and STOP the breakage! The Styling Spritz causes even more DRYNESS unless you use **ShamBOOsie's** secrets for avoiding the DRYNESS! In six to eight weeks you start the whole process over again; it never STOPS and they are making billions while you are becoming more and more like ShamBOOsie—**BALD**!

If something isn't done, over 85 percent of all black females in this country will be BALD by the end of the next Decade! The definition of the word *destruction* is **"The act of destroying or the condition of being destroyed, ruin, or a means or cause of destroying!"** All of this is associated with what is happening to the black female's hair, caused by the application of this Notorious Chemical, **Dehydrating Monster, the In-Home Chemical NO-Lye Relaxer KIT!** It robs the hair of its "Life" and "Body" and it's nearly impossible to remove this extremely **Dehydrating Monster!** It is Killing Black Hair.

For all black females that apply a **No-Lye Relaxer Kit**, it is nearly IMPOSSIBLE to reverse the effects on their hair. The Makers of these, substandard, shoddy, good for nothing **black hair products** are destroying your New GROWTH faster than you can GROW it.

The fact that you are putting a relaxer in your hair every time you turn around, says "Your HAIR is GROWING!" The average black woman who has never attended a Cosmetology School is self-applying one of the most dangerous, most destructive products ever made specifically for the hair of black women. There are so many things you don't know about this Chemical. For instance, did you know that this **"Hair Killer"** is made even with L'Oreal knowing the effect it will have on your HAIR?

The Hair Killing Kitchen Chemists

The Kitchen Chemists are those women standing in their kitchens and bathrooms combing this "hair killer" through your hair. Then after the hair you are GROWING and relaxing every six to eight weeks has been destroyed, you must spend your money to attach somebody else's hair to what little hair the Kitchen Chemist has left you with!

Chemically Relaxing **and** Coloring your Hair at Home is DANGEROUS! You need a one-on-one Hair Color Consultation with a professional; it is a must! Of course you can color your hair at home, but if you are new to hair color, I would highly recommend beginning the process with a one-on-one Hair Color Consultation with a professional. Also, you must take into consideration the other chemical, the relaxer, in your hair. Many of you think that hair color is not a chemical, but it is, and it will totally change the texture of your hair. If your select the wrong type of chemical, you can say "good-bye" to your hair.

Never Trust a **Hair Killing Kitchen Chemist;** she hasn't any idea of what she is doing. In fact don't trust Cathy either! Cathy is a **Hair Killing Kitchen Chemist.** She doesn't have a professional hair care license and has never been to a cosmetology school. Everything she has to say is the OPINION of someone else.

Just Do EXACTLY as this Book Says and Get the EXACT Results. Its methods are based on the Theory of Cosmetology and the Laws and Science of Trichology (the Study of Hair).

You Must CONDITION Your HAIR Every Time

- Did you ever wonder what actually happens in salons when you visit for service?
- Did you know that most salons will use a cheaper brand of shampoo and conditioner on your hair, but will sell you the better products for Conditioning Treatments at home?
- Did you know that when cheap conditioners are used on your hair, they actually damage the hair?
- Very often the products sold in the salon will not be the best products for your hair. They will not work no matter how much or how often you use them.
- You must answer the question what does the condition of your hair dictate?
- I choose the EXACT conditioning product for the hair at the time I'm servicing the hair, so that the hair gets what it needs.

The idea is to TREAT the hair with every application of shampoo and CONDITIONER. I make sure the products I use are the BEST and the EXACT products for the client's needs.

Hair GROWTH Is About the Science of Hair, Products, and Cosmetology

It's the concept every School of Cosmetology should be teaching, the method by which every Salon and Stylist should operate and it's the manner in which every Manufacturer of Hair CARE Products,

Formulate, Develop, Design, and Produce their products. It makes perfect sense that it should be what you must consider when chemically relaxing, coloring, take care of, and GROW your HAIR. I have done all of the work in studying the theory of Cosmetology and the Science and Chemistry of your HAIR for you; all you need to do is acquaint yourself with my research. I will teach you everything.

It is my mission to make the "Scientific Study" of your hair, using the theory of Cosmetology and the art of personal beautification, simple enough that it will provide you with a working knowledge of the laws pertaining to caring for your hair. My desire is to somehow persuade you to "CHANGE" the things you are personally doing that are destroying own hair. The larger Hair CARE companies, the Beauty Giants will hire several competent Scientists that will have the responsibility of creating their products; they are paid a lot of money to come up with inferior conditioners. I for one professionally speaking, don't believe the Beauty Giants care enough, to spend enough money necessary to ensure the quality and that their cheap hair products will work.

The Scientists and Chemists

The Major Manufacturers of Hair Care Products employ some of the best Chemists and Scientists to design and formulate their Product lines. The products you need to Fix the various Problems you are experiencing are those that are EXACT products. It's not about brand names or anything else. The perception that Nexxus Products are **white hair products** is ridiculous. Products should be judged by whether they work or not. You probably have an assortment of jars, bottles and tubes of different kinds of Hair Products, but none of them are working for you. I have always required my new clients to bring all of the products they have at home with them to the salon on their first visit.

A Real Time TRANSFORMATION

The thing to keep in mind is that if you are using a chemical Relaxer to straighten your hair, you **MUST** also use **"ONLY High-End Hair CARE and Conditioning Products.** Here is where using the term **white hair care products** is the only way to get you to understand. This means you **"MUST"** use the product you refer to as **white hair care products!** ShamBOOsie uses Humectress **Ultimate Moisturizing Conditioner,** and Therappe Shampoo from Nexxus Products. The reason is because it is the ONLY Conditioner that will reverse the impossible DRYNESS that is taking out your hair.

Sustainable Moisture!

Humectress for softness when there is a No-LYE Relaxer in your hair because **Humectress Ultimate Moisturizing Conditioner** is the only thing that will work. Humectress can enhance the condition of your hair, with an elevated level of moisturization; it is specially formulated with Vitamin E, Coconut Oil, and Honey Extract and provides nourishing moisture, leaving hair luxuriously soft, manageable, and full of luster. Keep in mind that the beauty giants makes BOTH the poor quality and the high quality products. It's just that one line of products they make primarily for white women and the other for use on black women's hair.

Dudley's Crème Press Hairdressing is necessary to protect the hair from flat irons, hot irons, and blow dryers. **Crème Press** will give your hair **Sustainable Moisture** to ensure the **SOFTNESS** in your hair all day, every day! ShamBOOsie will also use Keraphix Restorative Strengthening Conditioner, if there is NOT a No-LYE Relaxer in your hair. When the hair has been relaxed with a LYE Relaxer or if the hair is still natural, ShamBOOsie uses **Keraphix Restorative Strengthening Conditioner,** which is specially formulated with Collagen and Keratin Amino Acids and gently repairs damage. It will help achieve softer, stronger, healthier-looking hair from root to tip.

A ShamBOOsie Tip: If you should use Keraphix Restorative Strengthening Conditioner on hair that was relaxed with a No-LYE Relaxer Kit it will increase the percentage of dryness and hair break-age times 1,000 percent. **Crème Press Hair Dressing** and **Humectress Ultimate Moisturizing Conditioner** will give your hair **Sustainable Moisture!**

The Bag Lady

A young woman called me because she had purchased a copy of my first book and wanted to become a new client. I was working at a chain salon in the mall at the time. She lived in New York City. She didn't have a car, so her trip to the salon in New Jersey required taking 3 buses. But she scheduled her appointment and looked forward to it with great enthusiasm.

I explained to her that I require all new clients to bring all the products they have been using with them on their first visit. (I look at all of the products and throw everything that isn't any good in the garbage, and sell them new products that will work for them. I don't do this just to sell hair care products because that would be stealing from my clients, and God wouldn't appreciate me stealing from his people.) But I should not have told this particular client to bring her products.

This new client was traveling that day on buses with her elderly mother, She was about two hours late for her appointment because of the products she was bringing for me to look at. Most new clients will have four or five different products. Finally, the new client and her elderly mother walked in pushing a personal shopping cart. When I saw it, I assumed they had been shopping in the mall and had just lost track of time. Right away she asked if I wanted to see her products, but I told her to wait until I had finished her hair. By the way, her elderly mother was all over the salon, giving me instructions as to how to handle her daughter's hair, until I made her go into the seating area and have a seat. Her daughter kept asking me if I wanted to see her hair products, and I kept asking her to wait!

Finally I finished cutting and styling her hair, and sat down to take a look at the products. She reached into the shopping cart and pulled out two huge plastic bags filled with hair products; then she reached in and pulled out another six bags of products from that shopping cart. In fact the entire shopping cart was filled with bottles, jars and tubes of every type of hair product imaginable. I threw away three trashcans filled to the top with junk hair products. She had over a $1,000.00 worth of products in her shopping cart and some of it was very High-End, High Quality hair care products, but most of it was poor, low quality products, and none of it had worked for her! In the end, my wife and I drove The Bag Lady and her mother all the way home to New York City because they had had such a trying experience lugging that shopping cart filled with hair care products on three buses, and by that time they were completely exhausted! God will give the increase…

I will only use Hair-End products that work very well and do exactly what I need it to do. Each product I use in the salon and recommend my readers was handpicked for what it can do to make the hair as healthy as possible. I am meticulous, and will test every product 1,000 times before I will recommend it. This is the only way I can guarantee the results. You can trust my every word because I have prayed and asked God to increase my dream, which is to help my people, finally get things right.

More About Shamboosie…

From an early age, ShamBOOsie dreamed of becoming a famous singer, but later he accepted that God the Creator had something else in mind for his life—helping women of color and their daughters to GROW and have longer, healthier hair. It is his desire that black females everywhere become as lovely and as beautiful as possible. ShamBOOsie is revered by his peers in the National and International Hair Styling and Fashion arena. He has served as Artistic Director for several of Hype Hair Magazine's Annual Natural Beauty Contests.

ShamBOOsie's specialization is a SAFER, PAINLESS method of applying the **Chemical LYE Relaxer** that guarantees NO SCALP BURNS EVER! This revolutionary concept has been long-waited and is preferred by hairdressers who master this simple application technique. This NO SCALP BURNS concept is the solution to one of the biggest hair care concerns for black women who chemically relax their hair. Unfortunately, there is no standard chemical relaxer application method. Therefore, one thousand people and one thousand Hairdressers will apply the Chemical Relaxer one thousand different ways. This is not good and you get as many different results and degrees of damage. Hairdressers, all have only one thing on their mind, getting the hair straight and getting YOUR money. So your hair falls out because no one cared UNTIL NOW!

ShamBOOsie has been featured/quoted in the beauty industry media, and he continues to be a sought-after educator, consultant and trainer. ShamBOOsie's passion for beautiful healthy hair is further evidenced by his unique ability to select the perfect High-End Hair CARE products with "genuine healing properties" that are best suited for black HAIR. His forthcoming How-to-DVD's will demonstrate the total concept of ShamBOOsie's Hair Wellness Approach to Hair Growth.

Beautiful Black Hair

He says, "I am most serious and passionate about my Hair Wellness Approach to Hair GROWTH and Hair CARE, a professional yet simple concept that leads the way in solving many issues with black HAIR. The **"Healing Within"** concept is that process by which my Hair Wellness Approach will get you there."

Often called "The Gentle Giant," ShamBOOsie has a spellbinding stage presence, yet he is disarmingly honest and straightforward when you meet him in person. His humor, eloquence and show-manship shine through at hair shows and other public appearances.

Throughout his career, ShamBOOsie has worked with leading companies such as Clairol Professional, Dudley's Products, JC Penney Salons, and Hype Hair Magazine. He is a Certified Hair Instructor whose influence can be seen in his practical instructions, his proven philosophy of Salon services, and his commitment to beautiful healthy hair for women of color.

He remains at the forefront of the hairdressing industry because ShamBOOsie Knows and Understands black HAIR, and he expands his advisory role by hosting "Let's Talk Hair" seminars and by answering e-mail for women all over the world.

The Black Woman: God's Most Beautiful Creature

My absolute desire is to teach you everything you need to know with SIMPLICITY, to fill-in all the blanks, leaving no stone unturned. The most beautiful creature God has ever created is a **Black Woman**, and making a black woman's hair beautiful is my delight.

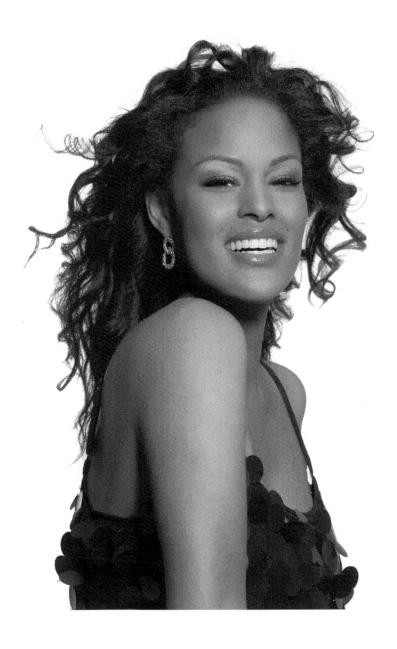

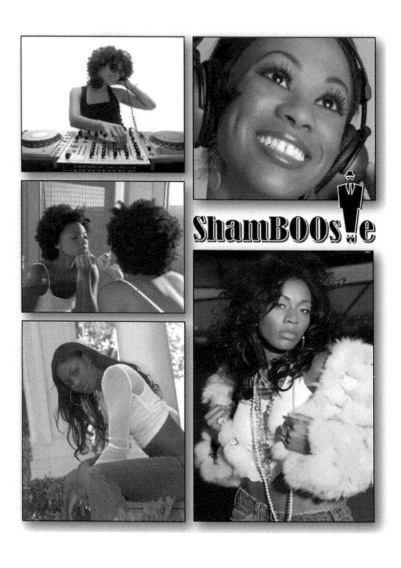

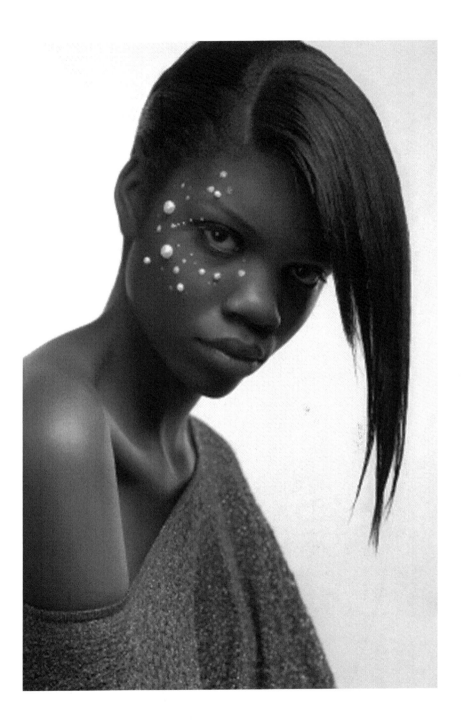

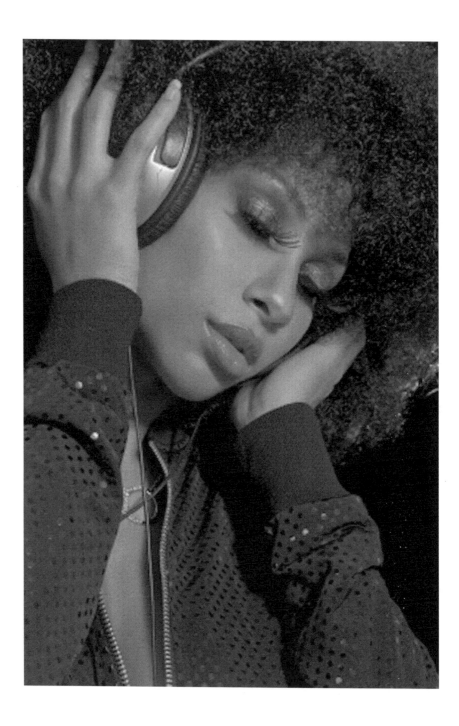

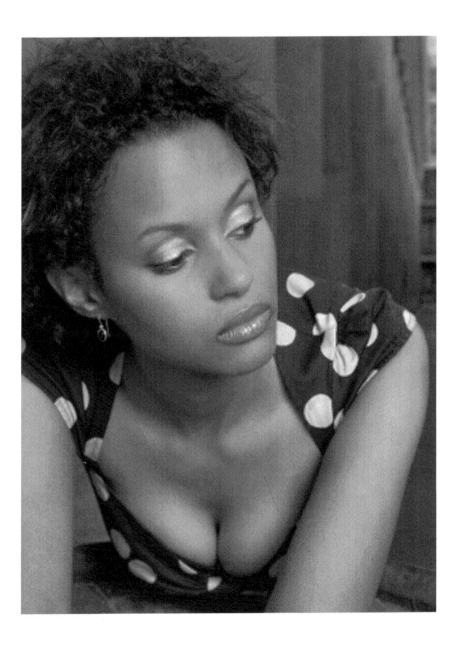

Beautiful Black Hair

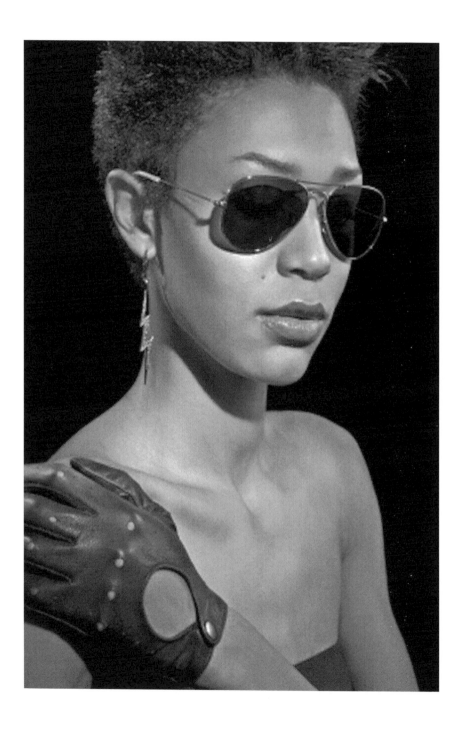

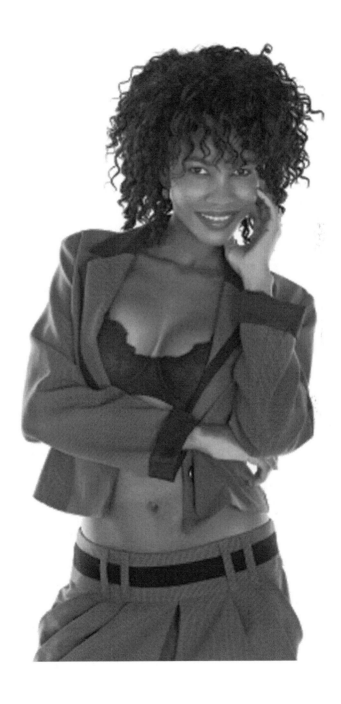

Beautiful Black Hair

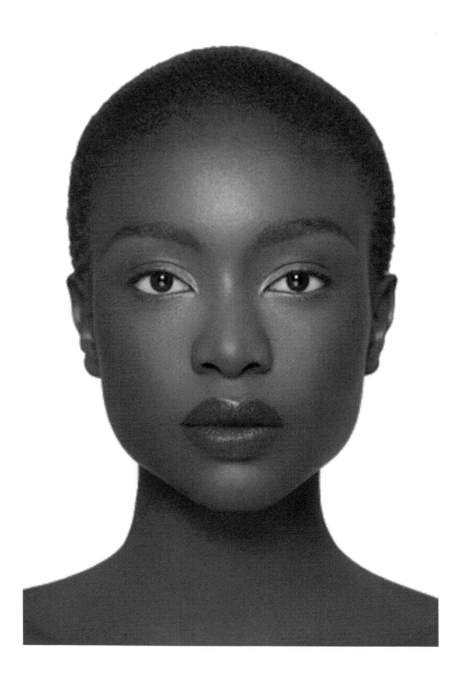

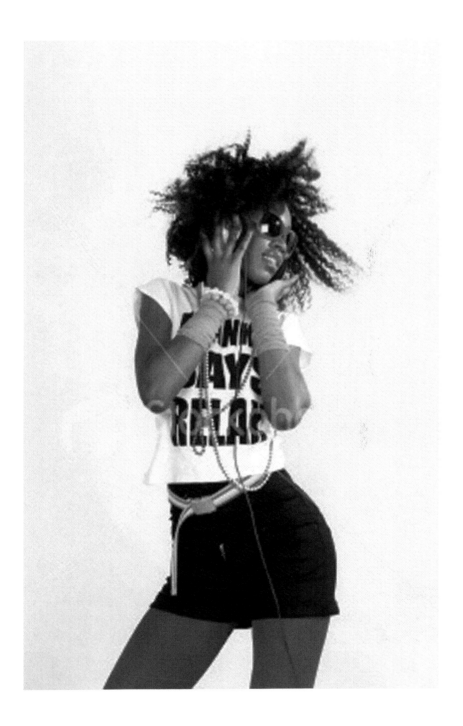

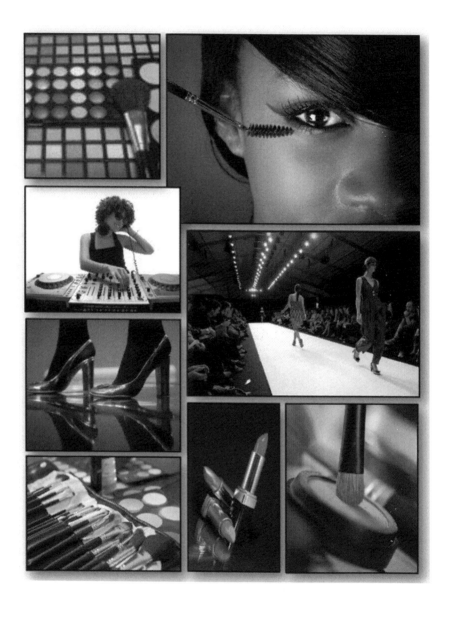

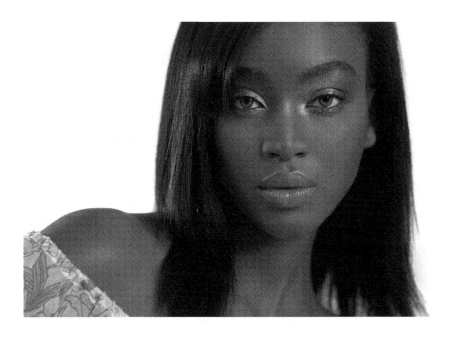

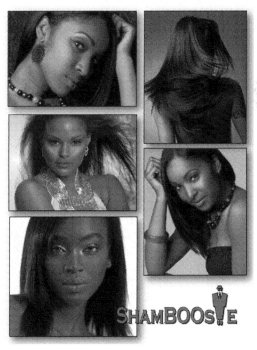

Glossary

1. Alkaline Perm:
A permanent wave product with a pH from 7.5 to 9.5, it is stronger, producing a more firm, springy curl.

2. Activator (for use with bleach)
Many times this product comes in a hair lightening kit, is used to speed up the action process of bleach also known as busters, accelerators, and lighteners. Activators do not increase the strength of lighteners and have little or no effect on the hair.

3. Ammonia:
This product in permanent hair color causes the developer to lighten the hair while at the same time enabling the color to be deposited. It is an alkaline found in hair color and is the ingredient that causes hair to become porous during the coloring process. When selecting a hair color for women of color, choose one free of ammonia.

4. Ammonium Thioglycolate:
Also known as (Thio) or (Curly Perm). It is an active chemical ingredient in permanent waves and ethnic curly perm products.

5. Basing Cream:
A protective oily cream that is applied to the scalp, ears, and neck before applying a relaxer or curling product to minimize the skin's contact with the chemical.

Beautiful Black Hair

6. Bonding:
Weaves, braids, and extensions are all methods of temporarily adding and attaching wefts, locks, or small sections of synthetic and human hair.

7. Bleach(ing):
Lighteners come in powder, cream, or gel form. This product chemically strips so much more than just color from the hair that, in many cases, it leaves black hair lifeless. It is very dangerous to apply other chemicals, such as relaxers, and Thio perms on top of bleach. There are many other safer ways to lighten the hair.

8. Clarifying Shampoo:
Used to remove most any type buildup on the hair. It cleans deeply because of its strong detergent base.

9. Color remover:
Designed for removing unwanted artificial hair color. There is a separate color remover for permanent and semi-permanent hair color.

10. Cool:
The colors blue, green, and violet-based tones in permanent hair color are referred to as cool. Their job is to enhance or neutralize unwanted tones when coloring hair.

11. Curl Activator and Moisturizer:
A maintenance product for chemically curled hair, used to soften, moisturize, and "revive" the curl.

12. Dandruff:
A white flaky buildup of dead skin cells found on both an oily scalp and a dry scalp, which means the flakes can be dry or oily.

13. Double Process:
Lightening the hair or changing the natural color with bleach, which is the first process, and toning or recoloring the hair with a new shade, which is the second process.

14. Elasticity:
The hair's ability to stretch without breaking and return to its original shape. The elasticity determines how well the hair will hold curl, which is an important factor in choosing the correct perms, color, and relaxers.

15. Hair Follicle:
An opening in the scalp through which a single shaft of hair grows.

16. Henna:
A hair dye that has been around for years but is still used today. Its name is derived from the plant from which it is made. This is an ancient Egyptian vegetable dye in powder form, which gives the hair reddish tones. It is metallic in nature, which means that once it is applied to the hair, this product will block any application of an ammonia/peroxide base hair color.

17. Hydrogen Peroxide:
A liquid or cream chemical developer when mixed with permanent hair color. It lifts the natural pigmentation of the hair, while at the same time, prepares the hair for the deposit of a new color. It also activates the lifting ingredient of powder, gel, and cream lightener.

18. Hairdressing:
The best hairdressing comes in the form of a light cream that conditions, moisturizes, and leaves the hair soft and silky to the touch, with

a slight sheen or shine. It can be used daily to dress the hair giving it a healthier appearance.

19. Grease:

Should be used lightly on the scalp and never on the hair. In some cases it may be used to base the scalp but only when manufactured for that purpose. Grease should never be used for dressing the hair because it is usually too oily.

20. Level or Level system:

All natural hair color falls within ten levels of shades, from black to lightest blond. Hair color manufacturers use the level system to chart their many different shades and colors, from warmest brown, red, and gold, to the coolest ash shades.

21. Lye:

The chemical ingredient used to formulate Sodium Hydroxide relaxers.

22. Low Lights:

After the hair has received as many highlights as possible, an opposite process of toning some strands of hair is referred to as low lighting. Usually hair colors mixed with ten-volume developer or semi-permanent hair colors are used for this purpose.

23. Melanin:

Microscopic granules filled with molecules of melanin. There are two types that make up the natural color of hair. Eumelanin makes the dark or black pigment in hair, and Pheomelanin, makes the red/yellow pigment in hair. A mixture of the two is called Mixed Melanin. If the hair has no color, it has no melanin.

24. Metallic Dye:
Hair dye that gets its color from metallic salts and from lead.

25. Neutralizer:
The chemical applied at the end of a curl or relaxer to completely stop the chemical process and return the hair to its normal pH level. Sold in clear liquids, creams, lotions, and shampoo form.

26. No-Lye Relaxer:
The common term for every chemical used to relax hair that contains (No-Lye) or no sodium hydroxide as its active chemical ingredient. The Calcium Hydroxide Relaxer (the BALD-faced LYE) is by far the most dangerous but the most widely used relaxer on the market today. This chemical is a HAIR KILLER!

Even if you use it only one time, you could lose all of your hair, so stay away from this one. It is a very different product from the Sodium Hydroxide Relaxer. Some others contain Ammonium Thioglycolate, Lithium Hydroxide, and Potassium Hydroxide.

27. Porosity:
The hair's ability to absorb moisture. When the hair is slightly porous, it is soft or moist, allowing chemical relaxer, hair color, and conditioners to ease their way through the cuticle layer, into the cortex layer of the hair. The NO-LYE relaxer restricts the hair's ability to absorb moisture by actually locking it out. This causes the hair to be very dry and promotes the possibility of breakage.

28. Protein:
A complex organic compound that contains amino acids as its basic structural units found in all living tissue, skin, hair, and nails. The hair is made up of about 98 percent protein, which is why there are

many protein treatments designed to rebuild strength in hair that has lost its elasticity by adding protein to the cortex.

Most black hair care products contain protein. If you always choose and use the best and highest quality of these products, they will give you the best chance for a healthy head of hair. Remember, there is no substitute for quality hair care products.

29. Over-processed hair:
Hair that is dry, brittle, and damaged from chemical. Many people do their own chemical services at home without a thorough knowledge of how the chemical process works. Also, most of the time people do not read or follow the instructions precisely.

Many times when the hair becomes over-processed from a hair color, perms, relaxers, and even conditioners. Some women have two to four chemicals in the hair at the same time, and each chemical is applied and over-processed. This kind of damage could be next to impossible to fix. Most of problems can be avoided by carefully reading and following the instructions.

30. Perm:
In the past, the relaxer was called a permanent (perm), meaning the hair has been permanently relaxed. Today, the term refers to Thio, short for Ammonium Thioglycolate, and the curly perm.

31. S Pattern:
A curly perm is wrapped on perm rods, and a few of them must be unrolled to check for a well-defined wave pattern, which is referred to as the S Pattern. Hair that is relaxed 80 percent or less with a lye relaxer is referred to as the S Curl.

32. Sodium Hydroxide:
A very high alkaline product used to permanently straighten hair. A Conditioning Lye Relaxer is the very best way to relax the hair. Buy and use only the very highest quality.

33. Setting Lotion:
A Medium hold product for hair that adds volume, shape and style and controls curls.

34. The pH:
The symbol for potential hydrogen concentration; the degree of acidity or alkalinity of any water-based solution. A pH of 7 is neutral, on a scale from 0 (very acidic) to 14 (very alkaline). Human hair seems to thrive best at 4.5 to 6.5, a slightly acidic pH level. Permanent hair coloring is an alkaline chemical process that temporarily raises the hair's pH to 10 or 11.

35. Processing Time:
The amount of time hair color, permanent waving solution, or relaxer remains on the hair before being rinsed out. The processing method is how the product works. Most perm products process at room temperature.

36. Resistant:
Hair that is very difficult to perm, chemically relax, or permanently color is called resistant. It means that the cuticle of the hair is very strong, and lies too flat and tightly against the hair shaft to allow moisture to enter. Many times the hair must be pre-softened to get the cuticle layer of the hair to open.

37. Warm:

The colors gold, orange, or red-based tones in permanent hair color are referred to as warm. Their job is to enhance or neutralize unwanted tones when coloring hair.

38. Weave:

A temporary way to add more hair to a person's real hair where strands of human or synthetic hair are sewn, bonded, or glued into place.

39. Weft:

A lock of human or synthetic hair used for weaving, extensions, and bonding.

40. Wrapping Lotion:

A setting lotion that is used for molding smoothly wrapped sets. Any setting lotion will do the same thing.

41. Virgin Hair:

Hair that has never been permed, colored, straightened or otherwise chemically treated.

If you have questions or comments, contact me:

shamboosie2@aol.com

Please know that in my heart the Lord God speaks to me constantly about the mission He has given me to accomplish, teaching every Black Woman and Black Mother and her daughters, as much about their hair as possible. So share what you learn from this book and tell everyone you know about these books.

ShamBOOsie

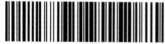

Made in the USA
Charleston, SC
06 April 2012